Number 297 ● April 16, 1998

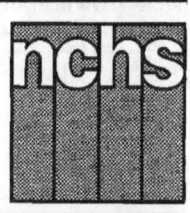

Advance Data

From Vital and Health Statistics of the CENTERS FOR DISEASE CONTROL AND PREVENTION/National Center for Health Statistics

An Overview of Home Health and Hospice Care Patients: 1996 National Home and Hospice Care Survey

by Barbara J. Haupt, D.V.M., Division of Health Care Statistics

Abstract

Objective—This report presents numbers and percents of home health and hospice care agencies, their current patients, and their discharges. Agency characteristics include type of ownership, region, certification, location, and affiliation. Patient and discharge characteristics include age, sex, race, marital status, admission diagnoses, and procedures.

Methods—The data used for this report are from the National Center for Health Statistics' 1996 National Home and Hospice Care Survey. This is a sample survey through which data are collected on the use of home health and hospice care agencies in the United States.

Results—During 1996, there were an estimated 2.5 million current patients and 8.2 million discharges from 13,500 home health and hospice care agencies in the United States. The agencies tended to be proprietary, certified by Medicare and Medicaid as a home health agency, and located in a metropolitan statistical area. Almost half were part of a chain or group of agencies. The home health and hospice care patients and discharges tended to be 65 years of age and over, female, white, and married or widowed. The most common diagnoses for home health care patients were diseases of the circulatory system, and the most common diagnoses for hospice care patients were malignant neoplasms. About a third of the home health care patients and about a fifth of the hospice care patients had a surgical or diagnostic procedure related to their admission for care. The most common procedures for home health care patients were operations on the musculoskeletal system, and for hospice care patients they were miscellaneous diagnostic and therapeutic procedures.

Keywords: National Home and Hospice Care Survey ● long-term care ● current patients ● discharges ● diagnoses ● surgical and diagnostic procedures

Introduction

This report presents statistics on an estimated 2.5 million current patients and 8.2 million discharges from 13,500 home health and hospice care agencies in the United States and is the fourth in a series of reports on home health and hospice care agencies and the people they serve (1–3). The data presented were collected through the 1996 National Home and Hospice Care Survey (NHHCS), a nationwide sample survey that was first conducted by the National Center for Health Statistics in 1992 (4–7). The NHHCS, a segment of the long-term care component of the National Health Care Survey (8), was developed in response to the rapid growth in the number of home health and hospice care agencies throughout the United States. This growth led to a need for information on the availability and utilization of services offered by these agencies. The NHHCS collects information about the agencies that provide hospice and home health care services, their current patients, and their discharges.

As shown in table 1, the number of agencies providing home health and hospice care services in the United States rose from 8,000 in 1992 to 13,500 in 1996. These agencies provided care to 1.3 million patients at the time of the survey in 1992, 2.0 million in 1994, and 2.5 million in 1996. There were 3.3 million discharges from these agencies in 1991–92, 5.6 million in 1993–94, and 8.2 million in 1995–96.

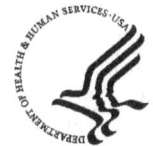

U.S. DEPARTMENT OF HEALTH AND HUMAN SERVICES
Centers for Disease Control and Prevention
National Center for Health Statistics

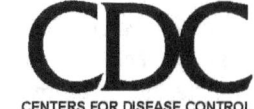

Table 1. Number of home health and hospice care agencies, current patients, and discharges: United States, 1992, 1994, and 1996

Type of estimate	1992	1994	1996
Agencies	8,000	10,900	13,500
Current patients	1,284,200	1,950,400	2,486,800
Discharges	3,273,300	5,600,200	8,168,900

Home health agencies and hospices are usually defined in terms of the type of care they provide. Home health care is provided to individuals and families in their place of residence to promote, maintain, or restore health or to maximize the level of independence while minimizing the effects of disability and illness, including terminal illness. Hospice care is defined as a program of palliative and supportive care services that provides physical, psychological, social, and spiritual care for dying persons, their families, and other loved ones. Hospice services, which are available in both the home and inpatient settings, may be provided by home health care agencies as well as by hospices.

Although this report provides some information about the agencies that provide home health and hospice care services, the focus of the report is the patients receiving the care. Patient estimates for current patients and for discharges are presented by agency and by demographic and diagnostic characteristics.

Methods

The 1,200 agencies included in the 1996 survey were selected from a universe of 16,700 agencies classified as agencies providing home health and hospice care. The universe was obtained from the 1991 National Health Provider Inventory (NHPI), updated to 1996 using the Agency Reporting System (9–11).

Data collection for the 1996 NHHCS was conducted between July and December 1996. Data were collected on a sample of current patients and of discharges from a representative sample of home health and hospice care agencies. Patient data were obtained from the medical records of the sampled patients and discharges. An overview of the data collection methods and

estimation procedures for the 1996 NHHCS is in the Technical Notes.

Statistics presented in this report are estimated numbers and percents of home health and hospice care agencies, current patients, and discharges by selected characteristics. Current patients are patients who were on the rolls of the agency as of midnight on the day immediately before the date of the survey. Discharges refer to patients who had been removed from the rolls of the agency (including those whose care ended because of death) during a designated month (from October 1995–September 1996) that was randomly selected for each agency.

Agency characteristics examined include ownership, Medicare and Medicaid certification, affiliation, and location. Ownership refers to the type of organization that controlled and operated the agency at the time of the survey. Affiliation refers to the agency's affiliation with a hospital, a group of agencies (such as a chain), a nursing home, or a health maintenance organization. Not all agencies are affiliated, and some may have other types of affiliation that are not included. Two types of location are reported: geographic region and metropolitan statistical area. Because of the dynamic nature of this area of the health care industry, an agency may provide home health care services, hospice care services, or both. Moreover, an agency may change its focus as the demand for different types of care changes. For this reason, data are not presented by type of agency, but by the type of care the patients were provided.

Patient information included in this report consists of selected demographic characteristics (sex, age, race, and marital status), diagnoses at admission, and surgical or diagnostic procedures related to the patient's admission to the agency. Diagnoses and procedures are coded according to the *International*

Classification of Diseases, 9th Revision, Clinical Modification (12).

The tests of significance used to test all comparisons mentioned in this report are based on the Bonferroni multiple comparisons using the z-test with an overall 0.05 level of significance. Not all differences were tested, so lack of comment in the text does not mean that the difference was not statistically significant. Estimates in this report have been rounded to the nearest hundred. Therefore, detailed figures may not add to totals. Percents were calculated using unrounded figures and may not agree with computations made from the rounded data.

Results

Agency Characteristics

In 1996, there were an estimated 13,500 home health and hospice care agencies providing services to patients in the United States (table 2). Thirty-four percent were owned by voluntary nonprofit organizations, 54 percent were proprietary or privately owned agencies, and 11 percent were owned by government and other agencies. Eighty-eight percent of the agencies were certified under Medicare (83 percent as a home health agency and 21 percent as a hospice), and 86 percent were certified under Medicaid (81 percent as a home health agency and 19 percent as a hospice). Eight percent of the agencies were not certified by either Medicare or Medicaid. Almost half—48 percent—of the agencies were part of a group or chain of agencies and 27 percent were operated by a hospital.

Forty percent of the agencies were located in the South region, 27 percent were in the Midwest, 18 percent were in the West, and 15 percent were in the Northeast. Two-thirds of the agencies were located in a metropolitan statistical area.

Table 3 provides information on current patients served by these agencies by the type of service provided (home health care or hospice care). At the time of the survey, there were a total of 2.5 million patients being served: 2.4 million (98 percent) were receiving home health care services and 59,400

Table 2. Number and percent distribution of home health and hospice care agencies by selected agency characteristics: United States, 1996

Agency characteristic	Number	Percent distribution
All agencies	13,500	100.0
Ownership		
Proprietary.	7,400	54.3
Voluntary nonprofit.	4,600	34.3
Government and other	1,500	11.4
Certification		
Certified by Medicare[1]	11,900	88.2
As a home health agency	11,300	83.4
As a hospice	2,900	21.3
Certified by Medicaid[1]	11,600	86.0
As a home health agency	11,000	81.4
As a hospice	2,600	18.9
Not certified	1,100	8.1
Affiliation		
Affiliated[1,2]	8,500	62.9
Part of group or chain	6,400	47.5
Operated by a hospital.	3,700	27.3
Not affiliated.	5,000	37.1
Geographic region		
Northeast	2,000	15.0
Midwest	3,700	27.0
South	5,400	40.1
West	2,400	18.0
Location of agency		
In a metropolitan statistical area	9,100	67.5
Not in a metropolitan statistical area	4,400	32.5

[1]Numbers may add to more than totals since an agency may be listed in more than one category.
[2]Includes a small number of agencies that are operated by a nursing home or a health maintenance organization.
NOTES: Numbers may not add to totals because of rounding. Percents are based on the unrounded figures.

(2 percent) were receiving hospice care services.

The ownership of agencies serving home health care patients differed significantly from those serving hospice care patients. Almost half of the home health care patients received care from voluntary nonprofit agencies and 42 percent were served by privately owned or proprietary agencies. On the other hand, the majority—85 percent —of hospice care patients were served by voluntary nonprofit agencies and 11 percent were served by proprietary agencies.

The majority of both home health and hospice care patients received services from agencies that were certified by Medicare and/or Medicaid. Forty-two percent were served by an agency that was part of a group or chain of agencies, and about a third were served by a hospital-affiliated agency. Although a larger percent of home

health care patients than of hospice care patients were served by a chain or a hospital-affiliated agency, the differences are not significant.

Of all the current patients, 33 percent were served by agencies in the South, 27 percent by agencies in the Midwest, 26 percent by agencies in the Northeast, and 14 percent by agencies in the West. Agencies that were located in an MSA served 80 percent of the patients.

The number and percent of discharges from home health and hospice care agencies are shown in table 4. As with current patients, the majority (60 percent) of the home health care discharges were from voluntary nonprofit agencies and 32 percent were from privately owned or proprietary agencies. The distribution of discharges from hospice care was also similar to that of current patients—85 percent were discharged from voluntary nonprofit

agencies and 13 percent by proprietary agencies. The majority of the discharges were from an agency that was certified under Medicare and/or Medicaid. Hospital-affiliated agencies had 47 percent of the discharges and agencies that were part of a group or chain of agencies had 39 percent of the discharges.

Of all the discharges, 30 percent were from agencies in the Northeast region, 25 percent were from agencies in the South, 24 percent were from agencies in the West, and 21 percent were from agencies in the Midwest. Eighty-eight percent of the discharges were from agencies located in an MSA.

Demographic Characteristics

Table 5 shows the number and percent of current home and hospice care patients by selected demographic characteristics. Two-thirds of the home health care patients and over half of the hospice care patients were female. Seventy-two percent of the patients receiving home health care services were elderly (65 years of age or older), 65 percent were white, 29 percent were married, and 35 percent were widowed. Of the hospice care patients, 78 percent were elderly, 84 percent were white, 44 percent were married, and 32 percent were widowed.

Table 6 presents the demographic information for home health and hospice care discharges. Sixty-four percent of the home health care discharges and 50 percent of the hospice care discharges were female. Two-thirds of the patients discharged from home health care services were elderly, 63 percent were white, 37 percent were married, and 25 percent were widowed. Of the hospice care discharges, 68 percent were elderly, 79 percent were white, 48 percent were married, and 29 percent were widowed.

Figure 1 shows that the reason for discharge from home health and from hospice care are very different. Almost 80 percent of the home health care patients were discharged because the services were no longer needed. Twenty-nine percent were discharged because they had recovered or their condition was stabilized, and 28 percent were discharged because their care was

Table 3. Number and percent distribution of home health and hospice care current patients by selected agency characteristics, according to type of care received: United States, 1996

Agency characteristic	All patients	Type of care		All patients	Type of care	
		Home health	Hospice		Home health	Hospice
		Number			Percent distribution	
Total.	2,486,800	2,427,500	59,400	100.0	100.0	100.0
Ownership						
Proprietary.	1,017,500	1,010,900	6,500	40.9	41.6	11.0
Voluntary nonprofit.	1,240,100	1,190,000	50,200	49.9	49.0	84.6
Government and other	229,200	226,600	*2,600	9.2	9.3	*4.4
Certification						
Certified by Medicare[1].	2,299,800	2,242,300	57,500	92.5	92.4	96.8
As a home health agency	2,259,300	2,229,700	29,600	90.9	91.9	49.8
As a hospice	652,100	596,000	56,100	26.2	24.6	94.4
Certified by Medicaid[1].	2,326,700	2,271,000	55,700	93.6	93.6	93.8
As a home health agency	2,293,700	2,264,800	28,800	92.2	93.3	48.6
As a hospice	579,200	526,600	52,600	23.3	21.7	88.5
Not certified	*104,300	*102,900	1,400	*4.2	*4.2	2.3
Affiliation						
Affiliated[1,2].	1,570,200	1,540,300	29,900	63.1	63.5	50.4
Part of group or chain	1,053,000	1,032,000	21,000	42.3	42.5	35.4
Operated by a hospital.	844,900	828,600	16,300	34.0	34.1	27.4
Not affiliated.	916,700	887,200	29,500	36.9	36.5	49.6
Geographic region						
Northeast	651,700	642,700	8,900	26.2	26.5	15.0
Midwest	668,100	646,900	21,300	26.9	26.6	35.9
South	811,300	792,300	19,000	32.6	32.6	32.0
West	355,700	345,600	10,100	14.3	14.2	17.1
Location of agency						
In a metropolitan statistical area	1,999,600	1,951,400	48,100	80.4	80.4	81.1
Not in a metropolitan statistical area	487,300	476,000	11,200	19.6	19.6	18.9

* Figure does not meet standard of reliability or precision.
[1]Numbers may add to more than totals since an agency may be listed in more than one category.
[2]Includes a small number of patients that were served by agencies that are operated by a nursing home or health maintenance organization.
NOTES: Numbers may not add to totals because of rounding. Percents are based on the unrounded figures.

being provided from another source (family or friends, transferred to another agency, or admitted to hospital inpatient services or a nursing home). Patients may also be enrolled in home health agencies in order to learn how to care for themselves. These patients have not recovered from their condition, but have learned how to cope with it so they can live independently. Twenty-one percent of the discharges no longer required services primarily for this reason. For hospice care patients, the reason for discharge for the majority (82 percent) was death, while 10 percent were discharged because their care was being provided by another source.

Diagnoses and Procedures

Information on the diagnoses of home health and hospice care patients was collected through the 1996 NHHCS. Up to six admission diagnoses were recorded for each patient. The number and percent of primary and all-listed diagnoses at admission are shown in table 7 for current patients, and similar information for discharges are shown in table 8. Home health care current patients had an average of 3.0 diagnoses per patient; for home health care discharges, there was an average of 2.7 diagnoses at admission. The average number of diagnoses at admission for hospice care patients was 2.5 for current patients and 2.2 for discharges.

The most common primary diagnosis for home health care current patients was a disease of the circulatory system—most often some form of heart disease. Other frequent primary diagnoses were diseases of the musculoskeletal system and connective tissue; diabetes mellitus; symptoms, signs, and ill-defined conditions; diseases of the respiratory system; and injury and poisoning. When looking at all-listed diagnoses, these same conditions also occurred most often. In addition, essential hypertension and diseases of the nervous system and sense organs were frequently listed secondary diagnoses.

As with current patients, the most common primary diagnosis for home health care discharges was a disease of the circulatory system—again, most often heart disease. Other frequent primary diagnoses were injury and poisoning (especially fractures, at 6 percent); malignant neoplasms;

Table 4. Number and percent distribution of home health and hospice care discharges by selected agency characteristics, according to type of care received: United States, 1995–96

Agency characteristic	All discharges	Type of care		All discharges	Type of care	
		Home health	Hospice		Home health	Hospice
	Number			Percent distribution		
Total.	8,168,900	7,775,700	393,200	100.0	100.0	100.0
Ownership						
Proprietary.	2,541,000	2,488,600	52,400	31.1	32.0	13.3
Voluntary nonprofit.	5,022,900	4,688,000	334,900	61.5	60.3	85.2
Government and other	605,100	599,200	*5,900	7.4	7.7	*1.5
Certification						
Certified by Medicare[1].	7,781,500	7,406,600	374,900	95.3	95.3	95.3
As a home health agency	7,573,200	7,370,500	202,700	92.7	94.8	51.6
As a hospice	2,477,700	2,119,100	358,600	30.3	27.3	91.2
Certified by Medicaid[1].	7,817,600	7,446,800	370,800	95.7	95.8	94.3
As a home health agency	7,642,400	7,430,100	212,300	93.6	95.6	54.0
As a hospice	2,265,300	1,932,000	333,300	27.7	24.8	84.8
Not certified	*181,100	*173,300	*7,800	*2.2	*2.2	*2.0
Affiliation						
Affiliated[1,2].	5,453,900	5,236,600	217,300	66.8	67.3	55.3
Part of a group or chain	3,145,500	3,012,700	132,700	38.5	38.7	33.8
Operated by a hospital.	3,832,000	3,708,300	123,700	46.9	47.7	31.5
Not affiliated.	2,715,000	2,539,100	175,900	33.2	32.7	44.7
Geographic region						
Northeast	2,422,700	2,351,100	71,700	29.7	30.2	18.2
Midwest	1,723,300	1,624,300	99,000	21.1	20.9	25.2
South	2,033,700	1,882,500	151,200	24.9	24.2	38.5
West	1,989,200	1,917,800	71,400	24.4	24.7	18.1
Location of agency						
In a metropolitan statistical area	7,216,800	6,885,600	331,300	88.3	88.6	84.2
Not in a metropolitan statistical area	952,100	890,100	62,000	11.7	11.4	15.8

* Figure does not meet standard of reliability or precision.

[1]Numbers may add to more than totals since an agency may be listed in more than one category.

[2]Includes a small number of discharges that were discharged from agencies that are operated by a nursing home or health maintenance organization.

NOTES: Numbers may not add to totals because of rounding. Percents are based on the unrounded figures.

diseases of the musculoskeletal system and connective tissue (especially arthropathies and related conditions, 4 percent); and diseases of the respiratory system (most often chronic obstructive pulmonary disease and allied conditions, 4 percent). When looking at all-listed diagnoses for home health care discharges, the most common diagnoses were diseases of the circulatory system, especially heart disease and essential hypertension. Other frequently listed secondary diagnoses were endocrine, nutritional, and metabolic diseases and immunity disorders, especially diabetes mellitus; and symptoms, signs, and ill-defined conditions.

The most common primary diagnosis for hospice care current patients was a malignant neoplasm (58 percent). Other frequent primary diagnoses included diseases of the circulatory system, diseases of the nervous system and sense organs, and diseases of the respiratory system. When looking at all-listed diagnoses, these same conditions also occurred frequently. In addition, endocrine, nutritional, and metabolic diseases and immunity disorders were frequently listed.

The most frequent primary admission diagnoses for hospice care discharges were malignant neoplasms (70 percent), diseases of the circulatory system (10 percent), and diseases of the respiratory system (5 percent). These were also the most common all-listed diagnoses.

In 1996, the NHHCS began collecting information on surgical or diagnostic procedures that were related to the patient's admission for care. Up to two procedures were recorded. Thirty-one percent, or 744,300 of the 2.4 million current home health care patients, had a surgical or diagnostic procedure related to their admission (table 9). These patients had 833,800 procedures, or an average of 1.1 procedures per patient. The most frequently performed procedures were operations on the musculoskeletal system, operations on the cardiovascular system, and miscellaneous diagnostic and therapeutic procedures.

Twenty-three percent, or 13,600 of the 59,400 hospice care current patients, had a procedure related to their

Table 5. Number and percent distribution of home health and hospice care current patients by age, sex, race, and marital status, according to type of care received: United States, 1996

Patient characteristic	All patients	Type of care		All patients	Type of care	
		Home health	Hospice		Home health	Hospice
		Number			Percent distribution	
Total.	2,486,800	2,427,500	59,400	100 0	100.0	100.0
Age at admission						
Under 45 years	351,700	347,400	4,300	14.1	14.3	7.3
45–54 years	132,900	130,200	2,700	5 3	5.4	4.5
55–64 years	193,800	187,600	6,100	7 8	7.7	10.3
65 years and over	1,799,500	1,753,400	46,100	72.4	72.2	77.7
65–69 years	218,600	213,600	5,000	8 8	8.8	8.4
70–74 years	323,900	314,300	9,600	13 0	12.9	16.2
75–79 years	426,000	416,200	9,800	17.1	17.1	16.6
80–84 years	413,400	404,300	9,100	16.6	16.7	15.2
85 years and over.	417,600	404,900	12,700	16 8	16.7	21.3
Unknown.	*	*	*	*	*	*
Sex						
Male	825,300	798,700	26,600	33 2	32.9	44.9
Female	1,661,200	1,628,500	32,700	66 8	67.1	55.1
Unknown.	*	*	*	*	*	*
Race						
White	1,629,000	1,579,300	49,700	65 5	65.1	83.7
Black and other.	342,300	336,600	5,700	13 8	13.9	9.6
Black.	297,400	292,400	4,900	12 0	12.0	8.3
Unknown.	515,600	511,500	4,000	20.7	21.1	6.7
Current marital status						
Married.	729,000	703,000	25,900	29 3	29.0	43.7
Widowed.	876,700	857,600	19,100	35 3	35.3	32.2
Divorced or separated.	105,700	100,100	5,500	4 2	4.1	9.3
Single or never married	460,200	455,100	5,000	18 5	18.7	8.5
Unknown.	315,400	311,600	*3,800	12.7	12.8	*6.3

* Figure does not meet standard of reliability or precision.

NOTES: Numbers may not add to totals because of rounding. Percents are based on the unrounded figures.

admission for care (table 9). These patients had 18,200 procedures, or an average of 1.3 procedures per patient. The most frequently performed procedures were miscellaneous diagnostic and therapeutic procedures and operations on the digestive system.

Information on discharges with a procedure related to admission is shown in table 10. Thirty-seven percent (2.9 million) of the 7.8 million discharges from home health care had a procedure. These discharges had 3,362,100 procedures, or an average of 1.2 procedures per discharge. The most common procedures were operations on the musculoskeletal system, operations on the cardiovascular system, and operations on the digestive system.

Hospice care discharges were similar to current hospice care patients regarding surgical and diagnostic procedures. That is, 21 percent (84,300) of the 393,200 discharges had an average of 1.3 procedures per discharge, for a total of 113,500 procedures. As with current hospice care patients, the most frequently reported procedures were miscellaneous diagnostic and therapeutic procedures and operations on the digestive system.

Summary and Discussion

The effort to control health care costs is one reason for the massive growth in the home health care industry. Home health care has reduced the number of hospital days in both terminally ill and nonterminally ill patients (13). Moreover, the increasing availability and use of home health care has mirrored the decreasing nursing

home occupancy rate (14) and the decreasing average length of stay in nursing homes (15). Because the average cost of a home care visit is considerably less than a day in a hospital or in a skilled long-term care facility (16), the growth in the home health care industry can be seen as a way to reduce health care costs. The steady increase in the elderly Medicare population of approximately 1.9 percent annually over the past decade is another major factor in the growth of the home health care industry (17). The use of the Medicare home health care benefit has increased dramatically since 1990; in 1995 Medicare home health care expenditures were almost 9 percent of total Medicare expenditures (18). The preference of the majority of the ever-increasing elderly population to recover

Table 6. Number and percent distribution of home health and hospice care discharges by age, sex, race, and marital status, according to type of care received: United States, 1995–96

Discharge characteristic	All discharges	Type of care		All discharges	Type of care	
		Home health	Hospice		Home health	Hospice
		Number			Percent distribution	
Total.	8,168,900	7,775,700	393,200	100.0	100.0	100.0
Age at admission						
Under 45 years.	1,549,800	1,518,100	31,700	19.0	19.5	8.1
45–54 years.	493,700	462,600	31,200	6.0	5.9	7.9
55–64 years.	710,500	652,400	58,200	8.7	8.4	14.8
65 years and over	5,402,700	5,137,500	265,200	66.1	66.1	67.5
65–69 years	874,500	840,400	34,100	10.7	10.8	8.7
70–74 years	1,085,900	1,024,600	61,300	13.3	13.2	15.6
75–79 years	1,024,400	967,400	57,000	12.5	12.4	14.5
80–84 years	1,152,600	1,104,300	48,300	14.1	14.2	12.3
85 years and over.	1,265,400	1,200,900	64,500	15.5	15.4	16.4
Unknown.	*	*	*	*	*	*
Sex						
Male	3,038,000	2,840,300	197,700	37.2	36.5	50.3
Female.	5,131,000	4,935,400	195,500	62.8	63.5	49.7
Race						
White	5,190,800	4,880,500	310,300	63.5	62.8	78.9
Black and other.	825,400	776,900	48,500	10.1	10.0	12.3
Black.	620,200	576,300	43,900	7.6	7.4	11.2
Unknown.	2,152,800	2,118,300	34,500	26.4	27.2	8.8
Marital status at discharge						
Married.	3,064,700	2,874,400	190,300	37.5	37.0	48.4
Widowed.	2,029,800	1,914,100	115,600	24.8	24.6	29.4
Divorced or separated.	411,400	385,900	25,500	5.0	5.0	6.5
Single or never married.	1,470,400	1,433,900	36,500	18.0	18.4	9.3
Unknown.	1,192,600	1,167,300	25,300	14.6	15.0	6.4

* Figure does not meet standard of reliability or precision.

NOTES: Numbers may not add to totals because of rounding. Percents are based on the unrounded figures.

from illness at home rather than in a hospital or nursing home is probably the major reason for this record growth.

Data from the NHHCS indicate that between 1992 and 1996, there was a 70 percent increase in the number of agencies providing home health and hospice care services in the United States. During this time, the number of current patients being served by these agencies increased 90 percent and the number of discharges more than doubled.

In 1996, an estimated 13,500 home health and hospice care agencies were providing services to 2.5 million patients in the United States and had 8.2 million discharges from care during the year. About a third of the agencies were owned by voluntary nonprofit organizations. These agencies served half of the patients and had 62 percent of the discharges. Almost 9 out of 10 of the agencies were certified under Medicare. However, about 30 percent of the patients and discharges were under 65 years old, indicating that these agencies provide services to a substantial number of the nonelderly as well as the elderly population.

The typical patient was an elderly white woman who was either married or widowed and was receiving home health care. Four out of 5 of the home health care patients were discharged from care because they no longer needed services. This included those who had recovered or whose condition had stabilized. Four out of 5 of the hospice care patients, on the other hand, were discharged because of death.

Comorbidity was common among both home health and hospice care patients—3 out of 4 of the home health care patients and discharges and 2 out of 3 of the hospice care patients and discharges had two or more diagnoses when they were admitted to the agency. Diseases of the circulatory system, diseases of the musculoskeletal system, and injury and poisoning accounted for over 40 percent of the diagnoses of home health care patients and discharges, while 60 percent of the hospice care patients and discharges had malignant neoplasms.

About a third of the current patients and discharges who received home health care had a surgical or diagnostic procedure related to their admission. Operations on the musculoskeletal system, operations on the cardiovascular system, and miscellaneous diagnostic and therapeutic procedures accounted for 2 out of 3 of the procedures performed.

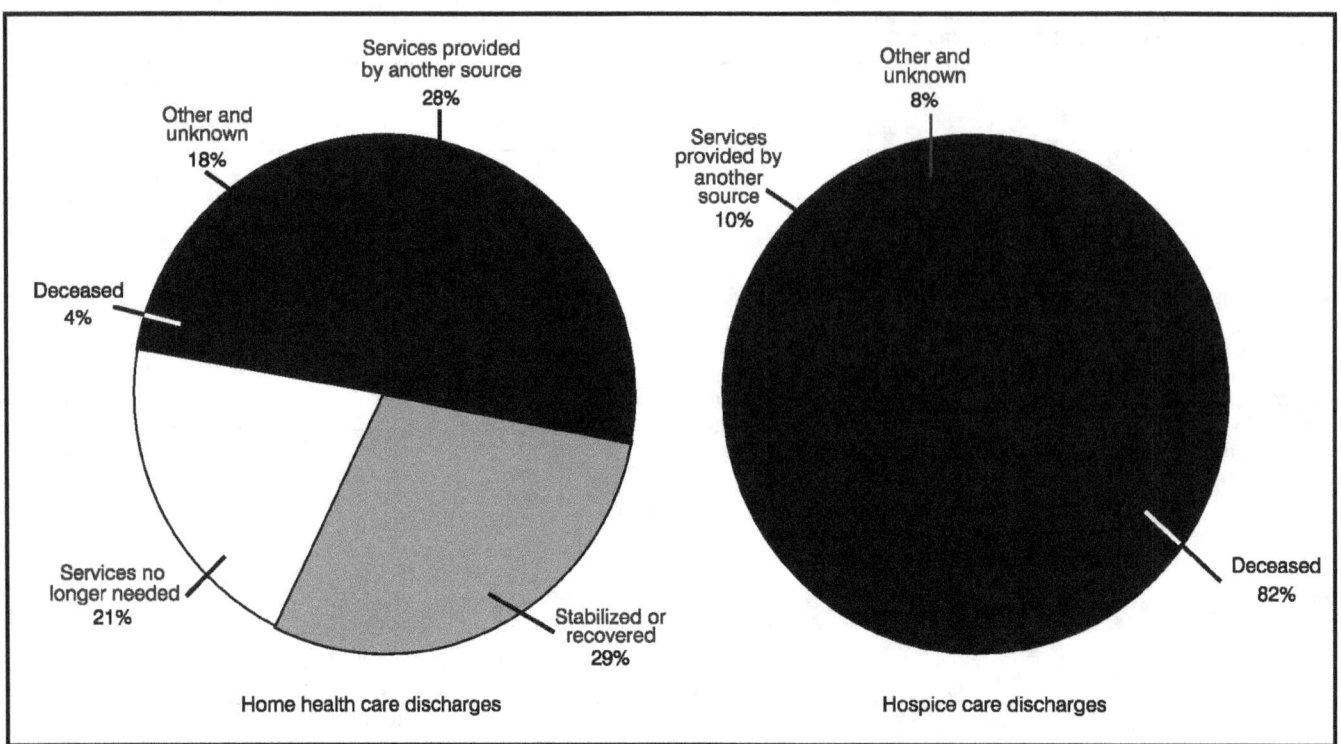

Home health care discharges

Hospice care discharges

Over one-fifth of the hospice care current patients and discharges had a procedure related to their admission for care. Miscellaneous diagnostic and therapeutic procedures and operations on the digestive system accounted for 9 out of 10 of the procedures for current patients and 8 out of 10 for discharges.

References

1. Strahan GW. Overview of home health and hospice care patients: Preliminary data from the 1992 National Home and Hospice Care Survey. Advance data from vital and health statistics; no. 235. Hyattsville, Maryland: National Center for Health Statistics. 1993.
2. Strahan GW. Overview of home health and hospice care patients: Preliminary data from the 1993 National Home and Hospice Care Survey. Advance data from vital and health statistics; no. 256. Hyattsville, Maryland: National Center for Health Statistics. 1994.
3. Strahan GW. An overview of home health and hospice care patients: 1994 National Home and Hospice Care Survey. Advance data from vital and health statistics; no. 274.

Hyattsville, Maryland: National Center for Health Statistics. 1996.
4. Haupt BJ. Development of the National Home and Hospice Care Survey. National Center for Health Statistics. Vital Health Stat. 1(33). 1994.
5. Haupt BJ, Hing E, Strahan G. The National Home and Hospice Care Survey: 1992 summary. National Center for Health Statistics. Vital Health Stat. 13(117). 1994.
6. Jones A, Strahan G. The National Home and Hospice Care Survey: 1993 summary. National Center for Health Statistics. Vital Health Stat. 13(123). 1996.
7. Jones A, Strahan G. The National Home and Hospice Care Survey: 1994 summary. National Center for Health Statistics. Vital Health Stat. 13(126). 1997.
8. Institute of Medicine. Toward a national health care survey, a data system for the 21st century. Washington: National Academy Press. 1992.
9. Delfosse R. Hospice and home health agency characteristics: United States, 1991. National Center for Health Statistics. Vital Health Stat. 13(120). 1995.
10. National Center for Health Statistics. Development and maintenance of a

national inventory of hospitals and institutions. National Center for Health Statistics. Vital Health Stat. 1(3). 1965.
11. National Center for Health Statistics. The Agency Reporting System for maintaining the national inventory of hospitals and institutions. National Center for Health Statistics. Vital Health Stat. 1(6). 1968.
12. Public Health Service and Health Care Financing Administration. International Classification of Diseases, 9th Revision, Clinical Modification. Washington: Public Health Service. 1991.
13. Hughes SL, et al. Impact of home care on hospital days: A meta analysis. HSR: Health Services Research. 32:4. October 1997.
14. Strahan GW. An overview of nursing homes and their current residents: Data from the 1995 National Nursing Home Survey. Advance data from vital and health statistics; no. 280. Hyattsville, Maryland: National Center for Health Statistics. 1997.
15. Dey A. Characteristics of elderly nursing home residents: Data from the 1995 National Nursing Home Survey. Advance data from vital and health statistics; no. 289. Hyattsville, Maryland: National Center for Health Statistics. 1997.

Table 7. Number and percent distribution of home health and hospice care current patients by first-listed and all-listed diagnoses at admission, according to type of care received: United States, 1996

	Primary diagnosis			All-listed diagnoses		
		Type of care			Type of care	
Admission diagnosis and ICD–9–CM code[1]	All patients	Home health	Hospice	All patients	Home health	Hospice
	Number					
Total.	2,486,800	2,427,500	59,400	7,138,400	7,171,500	146,900
Infectious and parasitic diseases 001–139	*19,200	*17,100	*2,100	52,800	48,300	4,500
Human immunodeficiency virus (HIV) disease 042	*5,100	*	*2,000	7,200	*	*2,000
Neoplasms. 140–239	162,100	126,800	35,400	278,300	221,800	56,500
Malignant neoplasms 140–208,230–234	149,600	115,000	34,600	259,000	203,700	55,300
Malignant neoplasm of trachea, bronchus, and lung 162,197.0,197.3	30,100	*	9,400	44,000	*32,400	11,600
Malignant neoplasm of breast 174–175,198.81	13,200	*	3,700	18,600	*14,700	3,900
Malignant neoplasm of prostate 185	10,700	*	3,900	18,600	*14,400	4,300
Endocrine, nutritional, and metabolic diseases and immunity disorders. . 240–279	247,400	247,200	*	802,500	795,100	7,300
Diabetes mellitus 250	203,700	203,600	*	548,300	545,200	3,200
Diseases of the blood and blood-forming organs 280–289	58,800	58,500	*	189,800	188,000	*1,900
Mental disorders 290–319	84,000	82,500	*	304,200	298,800	5,400
Diseases of the nervous system and sense organs. 320–389	144,100	139,300	4,800	462,400	453,700	8,800
Diseases of the circulatory system 390–459	623,000	615,700	7,300	2,099,500	2,071,000	28,600
Essential hypertension 401	107,500	107,500	*	604,100	599,800	4,200
Heart disease 391–392.0,393–398,402,404,410–416,420–429	267,700	262,800	4,900	884,400	868,400	16,000
Diseases of the respiratory system 460–519	190,500	186,200	4,400	463,500	453,700	9,800
Diseases of the digestive system 520–579	70,000	68,400	*1,500	263,100	258,600	4,500
Diseases of the genitourinary system 580–629	57,000	56,600	*	190,400	188,100	*2,400
Diseases of the skin and subcutaneous tissue. 680–709	85,900	85,900	*	170,000	169,400	*
Diseases of the musculoskeletal system and connective tissue 710–739	211,800	211,800	*	649,800	645,500	4,300
Symptoms, signs, and ill-defined conditions 780–799	196,100	194,800	*1,300	690,700	684,800	5,900
Injury and poisoning 800–999	166,800	166,800	*	292,800	291,800	*
Supplementary classification. V01–V82	88,500	88,400	*	286,000	280,700	5,300
All o her diagnoses 630–676,740–759,760–779	62,900	62,800	*	122,500	122,300	*
Unknown or no diagnosis.	*	*	–	. . .	. . .	. . .
	Percent distribution					
Total.	100.0	100.0	100.0	100.0	100.0	100 0
Infectious and parasitic diseases 001–139	*0.8	*0.7	*3.5	0.7	0.7	3.1
Human immunodeficiency virus (HIV) disease 042	*0.2	*	*3.3	0.1	*	*1.4
Neoplasms. 140–239	6.5	5.2	59.6	3.9	3.1	38.4
Malignant neoplasms 140–208,230–234	6.0	4.7	58.3	3.6	2.8	37.6
Malignant neoplasm of trachea, bronchus, and lung 162,197.0,197.3	1.2	*	15.8	0.6	*0.5	7 9
Malignant neoplasm of breast 174–175,198.81	0.5	*	6.2	0.3	*0.2	2.7
Malignant neoplasm of prostate 185	0.4	*	6.6	0.3	*0.2	2 9
Endocrine, nutritional, and metabolic diseases and immunity disorders. . 240–279	9.9	10.2	*	11.2	11.1	5.0
Diabetes mellitus 250	8.2	8.4	*	7.7	7.6	2.2
Diseases of the blood and blood-forming organs 280–289	2.4	2.4	*	2.7	2.6	*1 3
Mental disorders 290–319	3.4	3.4	*	4.3	4.2	3.7
Diseases of the nervous system and sense organs. 320–389	5.8	5.7	8.1	6.5	6.3	6 0
Diseases of the circulatory system 390–459	25.1	25.4	12.3	29.4	28.9	19.4
Essential hypertension 401	4.3	4.4	*	8.5	8.4	2.9
Heart disease 391–392.0,393–398,402,404,410–416,420–429	10.8	10.8	8.3	12.4	12.1	10.9
Diseases of the respiratory system 460–519	7.7	7.7	7.3	6.5	6.3	6.7
Diseases of the diges ive system 520–579	2.8	2.8	*2.5	3.7	3.6	3.1
Diseases of the genitourinary system 580–629	2.3	2.3	*	2.7	2.6	*1.6
Diseases of the skin and subcutaneous tissue. 680–709	3.5	3.5	*	2.4	2.4	*
Diseases of the musculoskeletal system and connective tissue 710–739	8.5	8.7	*	9.1	9.0	2 9
Symptoms, signs, and ill-defined conditions 780–799	7.9	8.0	*2.2	9.7	9.5	4 0
Injury and poisoning 800–999	6.7	6.9	*	4.1	4.1	*
Supplementary classification. V01–V82	3.6	3.6	*	4.0	3.9	3.6
All o her diagnoses 630–676,740–759,760–779	2.5	2.6	*	1.7	1.7	*
Unknown or no diagnosis.	*	*	–	. . .	. . .	. . .

* Figure does not meet standard of reliability or precision.

– Quantity zero.

. . . Category not applicable.

[1]Based on the *International Classification of Diseases, 9th Revision, Clinical Modification* (ICD–9–CM) (12).

NOTES: Numbers may not add to totals because of rounding. Percents are based on the unrounded figures.

Table 8. Number and percent distribution of home health and hospice care discharges by first-listed and all-listed diagnoses at admission, according to type of care received: United States, 1995–96

Admission diagnosis and ICD–9–CM code[1]	Primary diagnosis			All-listed diagnoses		
	All discharges	Type of care		All discharges	Type of care	
		Home health	Hospice		Home health	Hospice
	Number					
Total	8,168,900	7,775,700	393,200	21,953,900	21,089,100	864,800
Infectious and parasitic diseases . . . 001–139	166,400	*151,200	*15,200	385,700	362,500	*23,200
Human immunodeficiency virus (HIV) disease 042	*36,700	*	*11,500	*57,200	*	*13,800
Neoplasms . . . 140–239	948,200	670,700	277,500	1,661,300	1,228,800	432,500
Malignant neoplasms . . . 140–208,230–234	923,000	649,000	274,000	1,560,600	1,131,700	428,900
Malignant neoplasm of trachea, bronchus, and lung . . . 162,197.0,197.3	127,800	*41,700	86,000	213,800	110,000	103,800
Malignant neoplasm of breast . . . 174–175,198.81	*175,600	*	17,300	*233,300	*204,600	18,700
Malignant neoplasm of prostate 185	34,600	*	12,900	*82,700	*67,700	15,000
Endocrine, nutritional, and metabolic diseases and immunity disorders . . . 240–279	456,200	454,000	*	1,912,300	1,884,600	27,600
Diabetes mellitus 250	333,400	332,200	*	1,256,600	1,241,700	14,800
Diseases of the blood and blood-forming organs . . . 280–289	*130,500	*129,700	*	488,500	482,800	*5,700
Mental disorders . . . 290–319	138,800	133,800	*	728,400	707,000	21,400
Diseases of the nervous system and sense organs . . . 320–389	271,700	259,200	*12,500	870,800	836,300	34,500
Diseases of the circulatory system . . . 390–459	1,776,900	1,739,300	37,600	5,779,300	5,631,000	148,300
Essential hypertension 401	260,700	260,400	*	1,717,400	1,691,600	25,800
Heart disease . . . 391–392.0,393–398,402,404,410–416,420–429	999,100	972,100	26,900	2,884,400	2,810,300	74,100
Diseases of the respiratory system . . . 460–519	639,200	618,700	20,500	1,369,200	1,315,500	53,600
Diseases of the digestive system . . . 520–579	314,100	310,800	*	973,700	958,200	15,500
Diseases of the genitourinary system . . . 580–629	181,300	172,000	*9,300	711,100	692,600	18,500
Diseases of the skin and subcutaneous tissue . . . 680–709	190,100	189,400	*	421,800	417,200	*
Diseases of the musculoskeletal system and connective tissue . . . 710–739	629,200	628,300	*	1,617,600	1,600,700	*16,800
Symptoms, signs, and ill-defined conditions . . . 780–799	578,000	575,500	*	1,853,900	1,814,800	39,000
Injury and poisoning . . . 800–999	974,400	974,300	*	1,343,800	1,338,200	*
Supplementary classification . . . V01–V82	565,500	565,200	*	1,420,200	1,407,200	13,100
All o her diagnoses . . . 630–676,740–759,760–779	174,900	171,200	*	416,500	411,700	*
Unknown or no diagnosis . . .	*	*	*	. . .	. . .	. . .
	Percent distribution					
Total	100.0	100.0	100.0	100.0	100.0	100.0
Infectious and parasitic diseases . . . 001–139	2.0	*1.9	*3.9	1.8	1.7	*2.7
Human immunodeficiency virus (HIV) disease 042	*0.4	*	*2.9	*0.3	*	*1.6
Neoplasms . . . 140–239	11.6	8.6	70.6	7.6	5.8	50.0
Malignant neoplasms . . . 140–208,230–234	11.3	8.3	69.7	7.1	5.4	49.6
Malignant neoplasm of trachea, bronchus, and lung . . . 162,197.0,197.3	1.6	*0.5	21.9	1.0	0.5	12.0
Malignant neoplasm of breast . . . 174–175,198.81	*2.1	*	4.4	*1.0	*1.0	2.2
Malignant neoplasm of prostate 185	0.4	*	3.3	*0.4	*0.3	1.7
Endocrine, nutritional, and metabolic diseases and immunity disorders . . . 240–279	5.6	5.8	*	8.7	8.9	3.2
Diabetes mellitus 250	4.1	4.3	*	5.7	5.9	1.7
Diseases of the blood and blood-forming organs . . . 280–289	*1.6	*1.7	*	2.2	2.3	*0.7
Mental disorders . . . 290–319	1.7	1.7	*	3.3	3.4	2.5
Diseases of the nervous system and sense organs . . . 320–389	3.3	3.3	*3.2	4.0	4.0	4.0
Diseases of the circulatory system . . . 390–459	21.8	22.4	9.6	26.3	26.7	17.1
Essential hypertension 401	3.2	3.3	*	7.8	8.0	3.0
Heart disease . . . 391–392.0,393–398,402,404,410–416,420–429	12.2	12.5	6.8	13.1	13.3	8.6
Diseases of the respiratory system . . . 460–519	7.8	8.0	5.2	6.2	6.2	6.2
Diseases of the digestive system . . . 520–579	3.8	4.0	*	4.4	4.5	1.8
Diseases of the genitourinary system . . . 580–629	2.2	2.2	*2.4	3.2	3.3	2.1
Diseases of the skin and subcutaneous tissue . . . 680–709	2.3	2.4	*	1.9	2.0	*
Diseases of the musculoskeletal system and connective tissue . . . 710–739	7.7	8.1	*	7.4	7.6	*1.9
Symptoms, signs, and ill-defined conditions . . . 780–799	7.1	7.4	*	8.4	8.6	4.5
Injury and poisoning . . . 800–999	11.9	12.5	*	6.1	6.3	*
Supplementary classification . . . V01–V82	6.9	7.3	*	6.5	6.7	1.5
All o her diagnoses . . . 630–676,740–759,760–779	2.1	2.2	*	1.9	2.0	*
Unknown or no diagnosis . . .	*	*	*	. . .	. . .	. . .

* Figure does not meet standard of reliability or precision.

. . . Category not applicable.

[1] Based on the *International Classification of Diseases, 9th Revision, Clinical Modification* (ICD–9–CM) (12).

NOTES: Numbers may not add to totals because of rounding. Percents are based on the unrounded figures.

Table 9. Number and percent of current patients that had a surgical or diagnostic procedure related to admission for home health and hospice care by type of procedure and type of care received: United States, 1996

Procedure and ICD–9–CM code[1]	Total	Type of care	
		Home health	Hospice
	Number		
Patients with a procedure	757,900	744,300	13,600
	Percent		
Operations on the respiratory system 30–34	2.0	*1.8	10.1
Operations on the cardiovascular system 35–39	22.1	22.4	*
Operations on the heart and pericardium. 35–37	10.1	10.2	*
Operations on the digestive system 42–54	15.2	15.1	19.9
Operations on the intestines 45–46	4.9	4.8	*7.3
Operations on the musculoskeletal system 76–84	26.1	26.6	*
Reduction of fracture 76.7,79.0–79.3	7.2	7.3	*
Repair or replacement of hip 81.40,81.51–81.53	4.4	*4.4	*
Repair or replacement of knee 81.42–81.47,81.54–81.55	*6.1	*6.2	–
Operations on the integumentary system 85–86	6.7	6.6	*10.7
Miscellaneous diagnostic and therapeutic procedures 87–99	21.5	20.6	72.2
Diagnostic radiology and related techniques and radioisotope scan and func ion study . . 87–88,92.0–92.1	6.8	6.2	*38.9
Microscopic examination (laboratory tests). 90–91	6.2	6.2	*8.5
Therapeutic radiology and chemotherapy 92.2,99.25	*1.7	*	13.9
All o her procedures	18.9	19.0	13.7

* Figure does not meet standard of reliability or precision.
– Quantity zero.
[1]Based on the *International Classification of Diseases, 9th Revision, Clinical Modification* (ICD–9–CM) (12).
NOTES: Figures may add to more than totals because a patient may have had more than one procedure. Percents are based on the unrounded numbers.

Table 10. Number and percent of discharges that had a surgical or diagnostic procedure related to admission for home health and hospice care by type of procedure and type of care received: United States, 1995–96

Procedure and ICD–9–CM code[1]	Total	Type of care	
		Home health	Hospice
	Number		
Discharges with a procedure.	2,978,100	2,893,800	84,300
	Percent		
Operations on the respiratory system .30–34	4.9	*4.6	*13.9
Operations on the cardiovascular system 35–39	18.8	19.1	*
Operations on the heart and pericardium. 35–37	12.6	12.9	*
Operations on the digestive system .42–54	16.9	16.9	18.1
Operations on the intestines 45–46	*9.3	*9.4	*5.7
Operations on the musculoskeletal system 76–84	33.3	34.2	*
Reduction of fracture 76.7,79.0–79.3	8.5	8.7	*
Repair or replacement of hip 81.40,81.51–81.53	5.4	5.6	–
Repair or replacement of knee 81.42–81.47,81.54–81.55	9.7	10.0	–
Operations on the integumentary system 85–86	9.7	9.8	*
Miscellaneous diagnostic and therapeutic procedures 87–99	16.6	15.3	*61.4
Diagnostic radiology and related techniques and radioisotope scan and func ion study . . 87–88,92.0–92.1	6.5	*6.0	*22.9
Microscopic examination (laboratory tests). 90–91	*4.5	*4.0	*21.0
Therapeutic radiology and chemotherapy 92.2,99.25	*1.4	*	*4.8
All o her procedures	16.5	16.3	23.3

* Figure does not meet standard of reliability or precision.
– Quantity zero.
[1]Based on the *International Classification of Diseases, 9th Revision, Clinical Modification* (ICD–9–CM) (12).
NOTES: Figures may add to more than totals because a discharge may have had more than one procedure. Percents are based on the unrounded numbers.

16. National Association of Home Care. (February 1995). Basic statistics about home care. Home Care News. Washington. 1995.

17. Bishop C, Skwara KC. Recent growth of Medicare home health. Health Affairs. 95–110. Fall 1993.

18. Mauser E. Medicare home health initiative: Current activities and future directions. Health Care

Financing Review. 18(3), 275–291. Spring 1997.

19. Haupt BJ, Jones A. The National Home and Hospice Care Survey: 1996 summary. National Center for Health Statistics. Vital Health Stat. To be published.

20. Hoffman K. Specifications for selecting the agencies for the 1996 National Home and Hospice Care Survey. Unpublished memo. 1996.

21. Hoffman K. Specification of estimators for NHHCS. Unpublished memo. 1997.

22. Shah BV, Barnwell BG, Hunt PN, La Vange LM. SUDAAN User's Manual, Release 5.50. Research Triangle Institute, Research Triangle Park, NC. 1991.

23. Gousen S. Constructing Generalized Variance Functions for NHHCS - 1996. Unpublished memo. 1998.

24. Hansen MH, Hurwitz WN, Madow WG. Sample Survey Methods and Theory, Vol. I. New York: John Wiley and Sons. 1991.

25. Cochran WG. Sampling Techniques. New York: John Wiley and Sons. 1953.

Technical Notes

Although a detailed report has been published about the development and conduct of the survey (4), a brief description of the technical aspects of the NHHCS are presented in this report because some aspects of the survey have changed since that earlier report. The sample design was changed from a three-stage to a two-stage probability design, and the data collection forms were slightly modified. Copies of the data collection forms are included in this report (figures I–III) and a more detailed description of the 1996 NHHCS will be included in a future report (19).

Scope of the Survey

The sampling frame for the 1996 National Home and Hospice Care Survey (NHHCS) consisted of 16,700 agencies classified as agencies providing home health and hospice care. These agencies were identified through the 1991 National Health Provider Inventory (NHPI), updated to 1996 using the Agency Reporting System (9–11). The NHPI is a comprehensive census of nursing and related care homes, residential care homes, home health care agencies, and hospices. It is conducted periodically by NCHS. The sample consisted of 1,200 agencies selected from this universe.

Only agencies providing home health or hospice care services at the time of the survey were eligible to participate in the 1996 NHHCS. Of the 1,200 agencies in the sample, 1,091 were considered in scope of the survey. Of the 109 out-of-scope agencies, 89 were not providing home health or hospice care services at the time of the survey and 20 were duplicates or had merged with other sampled agencies. Of the in-scope agencies, 1,053 (97 percent) agreed to participate in the 1996 NHHCS, 34 refused to participate, and 3 could not be located.

Sampling Design

The sample design for the 1996 NHHCS was a stratified two-stage probability design (20). The first stage consisted of selecting a stratified sample of agencies. Each agency was placed into 1 of 24 strata based on type of agency (home health agency, hospice, or mixed agency), metropolitan statistical area (MSA) status (has an MSA code versus has no code), and region (Northeast, Midwest, South, and West). MSA is defined by the U.S. Office of Management and Budget on the basis of the 1980 Census. Within these sampling strata, agencies were arrayed by four types of ownership (profit, nonprofit, government, and unknown), three types of certification status (certified by Medicare and/or Medicaid, not certified, and unknown), State, MSA code, county, zip code, and size (number of current patients).

The second stage of sample selection, sampling of six current patients and six discharges within each agency, was done using a sample selection table to obtain systematic probability samples of current patients and of discharges. The patients and discharges were selected from lists constructed for each agency at the time of the interview. Current patients were defined as those patients who were on the rolls of the agency as of midnight on the day immediately before the date of the survey. Discharges referred to those patients who were discharged from care by the home health agency or hospice during a designated month between October 1995 and September 1996. Discharges that occurred because of death were included.

Data Collection and Processing

Data collection for the 1996 NHHCS began with a letter sent to all sampled agencies informing the administrator of the authorizing legislation, purpose, and content of the survey. Each agency was then contacted by an interviewer to discuss the survey and to arrange an appointment with the administrator.

Three questionnaires and two sampling lists were used to collect the data. The Agency Questionnaire was completed with the administrator or a person designated by the administrator. The interviewer then constructed the Current Patient Sampling List and the Discharged Patient Sampling List. These lists were used to select the sample patients and discharges. Sampling was accomplished by using tables showing sets of sample line numbers for each possible count of current patients and discharges in the agency. Up to six current patients and six discharges were selected.

After the samples had been selected, the Current Patient Questionnaires and the Discharged Patient Questionnaires were completed for each sampled person by interviewing the staff member most familiar with the care provided to the patient. The respondent referred to patient medical and other records as necessary. No patient was interviewed directly.

After the data had been collected, it was converted into machine-readable form by NCHS. Extensive editing was then conducted by computer to ensure that all responses were accurate, consistent, logical, and complete. The medical information recorded on the patient questionnaires was coded by NCHS staff according to the *International Classification of Diseases, 9th Revision, Clinical Modification* (12). Up to 12 diagnostic codes (a maximum of six at admission, and a maximum of six at the time of survey or discharge) and up to two procedure codes were assigned for each sample patient or discharge.

Estimation Procedures

Statistics presented in this report were derived by a multistage estimation procedure (21) that produces essentially unbiased national estimates and has three principal components. The first component, inflation by the reciprocals of the probabilities of sample selection, is the basic inflation weight. This component consists of the inverse of the probability of selecting the agency and the patient or discharge within each agency. The second component, which consists of an adjustment for nonresponse, brings estimates based only on the responding cases up to the level that would have been achieved if all eligible cases had responded. The third component, ratio adjustment to fixed totals, adjusts for over- or undersampling of agencies reported in the sampling frame.

Reliability of Estimates

Because the statistics presented in this report are based on a sample, they will differ somewhat from figures that would have been obtained if a complete census had been taken using the same schedules, instructions, and procedures. The standard error (SE) is primarily a measure of the variability that occurs by chance because a sample, rather than the entire universe, is surveyed. The SE also reflects part of the measurement error, but it does not measure any systematic biases in the data. The chances are about 95 in 100 that an estimate from the sample differs from the value that would be obtained from a complete census by less than twice the SE. However, SE's typically underestimate the true errors of the statistics because they reflect only errors due to sampling.

The SE's used in this report were approximated using SUDAAN software. SUDAAN computes SE's by using a first-order Taylor approximation of the deviation of estimates from their expected values. A description of the software and the approach it uses has been published (22). Although exact SE

Table I. Parameters used to compute standard error of numbers by type of estimate

Type of estimate	Parameters	
	A	B
Agency	0.019261	4.425270
Home health care		
Current patient	0.115800	1,328.865818
Discharge	0.265410	4,886.944977
Hospice care		
Current patient	0.018098	97.086178
Discharge	0.026362	432.006607

estimates were used in tests of significance in this report, SE's for aggregate estimates presented may be estimated using the general formula:

$$SE(X) = X \cdot RSE(X)$$

where X is the estimate and $RSE(X)$ is the relative standard error of the estimate. The relative standard error $(RSE(X))$ may be estimated using the following general formula (23):

$$RSE(X) = \sqrt{A + \frac{B}{X}}$$

where X is the estimate and A and B are the appropriate coefficients from table I.

To approximate the relative standard error $(RSE(p))$ and the standard error $(SE(p))$ of a percent p, the appropriate value of parameter B from table I is used in the following equation:

$$RSE(p) = \sqrt{\frac{B \cdot (1 - p)}{p \cdot y}}$$

where $p = 100 \cdot X/Y$, $X =$ the numerator of the estimated percent, and $Y =$ the denominator of the estimated percent and

$$SE(p) = p \ z \ RSE(p)$$

The standard error of a percent is valid only when one of the following conditions is satisfied: the relative standard error of the denominator is 5 percent or less (24) or the relative standard errors of the numerator and the denominator are both 10 percent or less (25).

Presentation of Estimates

Publication of estimates for the NHHCS is based on the RSE of the

estimate and the number of sample records on which the estimate is based (referred to as the sample size). Estimates are not presented in NCHS reports unless a reasonable assumption regarding the probability distribution of the sampling error is possible.

Because of the complex sample design of the NHHCS, the following guidelines are used for presenting the estimates:

If the sample size is less than 30, the value of the estimate is not reported.

If the sample size is 30–59, or if the sample is 60 or more and the RSE is 30 percent or more, the estimate is reported but should not be assumed reliable. This is indicated by an asterisk (*) in the tables.

If the sample size is 60 or more and the RSE is less than 30 percent, the estimate is reported and is considered reliable.

OMB No. 0920-0298: Approval Expires 03/31/97

FORM **HHCS-1**
(3-29-96)

U.S. DEPARTMENT OF COMMERCE
BUREAU OF THE CENSUS
ACTING AS COLLECTING AGENT FOR THE
DEPARTMENT OF HEALTH AND HUMAN SERVICES
U.S. PUBLIC HEALTH SERVICE
CENTERS FOR DISEASE CONTROL AND PREVENTION
NATIONAL CENTER FOR HEALTH STATISTICS

AGENCY QUESTIONNAIRE

1996 NATIONAL HOME AND HOSPICE CARE SURVEY

NOTICE – Public reporting burden for this collection of information is estimated to average 20 minutes per response, including the time for reviewing instructions, searching existing data sources, gathering and maintaining the data needed, and completing and reviewing the collection of information. Send comments regarding this burden estimate or any other aspect of this collection of information, including suggestions for reducing this burden to DHHS Reports Clearance Officer; Paperwork Reduction Project (0920-0298) Room 531-H; Hubert H. Humphrey Bldg.; 200 Independence Ave., SW; Washington, DC 20201. Information contained on this form which would permit identification of any individual or establishment has been collected with a guarantee that it will be held in strict confidence, will be used for purposes stated for this study, and will not be disclosed or released to others without the consent of the individual or establishment in accordance with Section 308(d) of the Public Health Service Act (42 USC 242m).

Section A – AGENCY INFORMATION

1a. Agency telephone number

b. Alternate telephone number

c. Alternate telephone number

2a. Administrator name

b. Respondent name

Notes

Section B – RECORD OF CONTACTS

Day (a)	Date (b)	Time (c)	Notes (d)
		a.m. / p.m.	
		a.m. / p.m.	
		a.m. / p.m.	
		a.m. / p.m.	
		a.m. / p.m.	
		a.m. / p.m.	
		a.m. / p.m.	
		a.m. / p.m.	
		a.m. / p.m.	

Section C – RECORD OF INTERVIEW

1. STATUS OF INTERVIEW – *Mark (X) appropriate box.*
   - 01 ☐ Complete interview
   - 02 ☐ Partial interview
   - 03 ☐ Refusal
   - 04 ☐ Unable to locate
   - 05 ☐ Not a Hospice/Home Health Agency
   - 06 ☐ Temporarily closed
   - 07 ☐ Not yet in operation
   - 08 ☐ No longer operating
   - 09 ☐ Merged with (Control No.) _____
   - 10 ☐ Duplicate (Control No. of duplicate) _____
   - 11 ☐ Other noninterview – *Specify* _____

2. Date of interview

Month	Day	Year

3. Field Representative name | FR Code

Figure I. Agency Questionnaire

Section D – ARRANGING THE ADMINISTRATOR APPOINTMENT

1. INTRODUCTION

Good morning (afternoon). My name is . . .. I'm from the Bureau of the Census. We are currently conducting the National Home and Hospice Care Survey for the National Center for Health Statistics which is part of the Centers for Disease Control and Prevention. We are studying home health agencies, hospices and their patients. You should have received a letter from Mr. John Anderson, the Acting Director of the National Center for Health Statistics, which describes this project. Have you received this letter?

☐ Yes – *Skip to Item 3 , NAME VERIFICATION.*
☐ No – *Continue with Item 2, SURVEY EXPLANATION.*

2. SURVEY EXPLANATION

If administrator wants a copy of the letter, explain that you will bring a copy when you visit the agency.

I'm sorry that you did not receive the letter. Let me briefly outline its contents.

The National Home and Hospice Care Survey is authorized under Section 306 of the Public Health Service Act to collect information about home and hospice care agencies, their services, and patients. The survey is endorsed by the National Association for Home Care and the National Hospice Organization. The statistics compiled from the data are used to support research for effective treatment of long-term health problems and to study utilization of hospice and home care agencies and the efficient use of the Nation's health care resources.

All information which would permit identification of the individual patient or agency will be held in strict confidence, will be used ONLY by persons involved in the survey and only for the purposes of the survey, and will not be disclosed or released to others for any purpose.

The survey includes a small sample of hospices and home health agencies. Although your participation is voluntary and there are no penalties for refusing to answer any questions, it is essential that we obtain data from all sample agencies.

READ IF NECESSARY:

We are asking participants for a list of current patients and a list of discharges during a designated one-month period. We will draw a sample of 6 current patients and a sample of 6 discharges from the lists and complete a questionnaire for each of the 12 sampled patients.

Continue with Item 3, NAME VERIFICATION.

3. NAME VERIFICATION

I would like to verify some information from my records. Is *(Name of agency on label)* the correct name of your agency?

☐ Yes – *Go to Item 4, ADDRESS VERIFICATION*
☐ No – *Enter correct agency name below.*↙

[ ]

4. ADDRESS VERIFICATION

Is *(Address of agency on label)* the correct address?

☐ Yes – *Go to Item 5 – SET APPOINTMENT*
☐ No – *Enter correct agency address below.* ↙

Number Street		P.O. Box, Route, etc.
City or town		
State		ZIP Code

5. SET APPOINTMENT

I would like to arrange a morning appointment at your convenience to conduct the survey. What would be a convenient date and time to visit your agency?

Day	Date	Time	a.m. p.m.

Day	Date	Time	a.m. p.m.

6. Could you give me directions to your agency from some easy to identify starting point? *(Record directions in number 7 below.)*

Thank you very much for your time. I will see you at *(Time)* on *(Date)*. Good-bye.

7. DIRECTIONS TO AGENCY *(If needed)*

Section E – QUESTIONS ABOUT THE AGENCY

Before I begin the interview, I'd like to take a moment to explain the purpose of the survey. I believe you (received/did not receive) the letter from the National Center for Health Statistics.

If administrator did not receive the letter, hand him/her a copy. Allow him/her to briefly read it through.

As it says in the letter, the purpose of the National Home and Hospice Care Survey is to collect information about hospices and home health agencies such as yours. The information you provide is strictly confidential and will be used only by persons involved in the survey and only for the purposes of the survey.

HAND FLASHCARD 1

1a. What is the type of ownership of this agency as shown on this card?

Mark (X) only ONE box.

01 ☐ PROPRIETARY – Includes individual or private, partnership, corporation

02 ☐ NONPROFIT – Includes church-related, nonprofit corporation, other nonprofit ownership

03 ☐ STATE OR LOCAL GOVERNMENT – Includes State, county, city, city-county, hospital district or authority

04 ☐ FEDERAL GOVERNMENT – Includes USPHS, Armed Forces, Veterans Administration

05 ☐ Other – *Specify* ↙

_____

_____

b. Does this agency operate under the general authority of a hospital?

01 ☐ Yes
02 ☐ No

FORM HHCS-1 (3-29-96)

Figure I. Agency Questionnaire—Con.

Section E – QUESTIONS ABOUT THE AGENCY – Continued	
1c. Does this agency operate under the general authority of a nursing home?	01 ☐ Yes 02 ☐ No
d. Is *(Name of agency)* a member of a group of agencies operating under one corporate authority or corporate ownership?	01 ☐ Yes 02 ☐ No
2. Does this agency operate under the authority of a Health Maintenance Organization (HMO)?	01 ☐ Yes 02 ☐ No
3a. Is this agency certified under Medicare as a Home Health Agency?	01 ☐ Yes 02 ☐ No 03 ☐ Certification pending
b. Is this agency certified under Medicare as a Hospice?	01 ☐ Yes 02 ☐ No 03 ☐ Certification pending
4a. Is this agency certified under Medicaid as a Home Health Agency?	01 ☐ Yes 02 ☐ No 03 ☐ Certification pending
b. Is this agency certified under Medicaid as a Hospice?	01 ☐ Yes 02 ☐ No 03 ☐ Certification pending
5a. Does this agency provide bereavement care to families of the patients that you serve?	01 ☐ Yes 02 ☐ No
b. Does this agency provide pastoral care?	01 ☐ Yes 02 ☐ No
HAND FLASHCARD 2 **6.** Does this agency provide any of the following services? *Mark (X) all that apply.* *Probe:* **Any other services?**	00 ☐ None 01 ☐ Continuous home care 02 ☐ Counseling 03 ☐ Dental treatment services 04 ☐ Dietary and nutritional services 05 ☐ Durable medical equipment and supplies 06 ☐ Enterostomal therapy 07 ☐ High tech care (e.g., IV therapy) 08 ☐ Homemaker/Companion services 09 ☐ Meals on Wheels 10 ☐ Medications 11 ☐ Occupational therapy/Vocational therapy 12 ☐ Oral hygiene/Prevention services 13 ☐ Personal care 14 ☐ Physical therapy 15 ☐ Physician services 16 ☐ Referral services 17 ☐ Respite care (inpatient) 18 ☐ Skilled nursing services 19 ☐ Social Services 20 ☐ Speech therapy/Audiology 21 ☐ Spiritual care 22 ☐ Transportation 23 ☐ Volunteers 24 ☐ Other services – *Specify* ↗ _____
7a. Does this agency currently have any active patients?	01 ☐ Yes – *GO to item 7b* 02 ☐ No – *THANK THE RESPONDENT, END THE INTERVIEW, AND MARK CODE 11 IN SECTION C ON THE COVER PAGE.*
b. What is the number of your current active patients?	_____ . __ Number of patients 99999 ☐ Don't know
8a. What is the number of home health care patients currently being served by this agency?	_____ Number of home health patients 0000 ☐ None 99999 ☐ Don't know
b. What is the number of hospice care patients currently being served by this agency?	_____ Number of hospice patients 0000 ☐ None 99999 ☐ Don't know

Figure I. Agency Questionnaire—Con.

Section E – QUESTIONS ABOUT THE AGENCY – Continued

READT ▶ To complete this survey, I will need a list of all current home health and hospice patients, and a list of all home health and hospice discharges for the month of *(Insert discharge sample month and year).*

From these lists, I will draw a sample of up to 6 current patients and up to 6 discharges.

9a. **From whom shall I obtain the list of current patients?**	Name
	Title
I will need these patients' medical records and the cooperation of a staff member best acquainted with these patients in order to obtain the information on this questionnaire.	
Hand the administrator a copy of the current patient questionnaire. Allow him/her to examine it briefly. Retrieve the questionnaire and continue reading.	01 ☐ Yes – *GO to item 10a* 02 ☐ No – *Determine which staff member would have this knowledge and enter the name and title below.* ↙
I will not be contacting or interviewing the patients in any way. I will depend on your staff to consult the medical records.	Name
b. **Would** *(person named in item 9a)* **know which staff member I should interview for those patients selected for the sample?**	Title
10a. **From whom shall I obtain the list of discharges?**	☐ Same as 9a
	Name
	Title
I will need the help of a staff person familiar with the discharge records to aid me in completing the information requested in this questionnaire.	
Hand the administrator a copy of the discharged patient questionnaire. Allow him/her to examine it briefly. Retrieve the questionnaire and continue reading.	01 ☐ Yes – *GO to item 11 below* 02 ☐ No – *Determine which staff member would have this knowledge and enter the name and title below.* ↙
	Name
b. **Would** *(person named in item 10a)* **know which staff member I should interview for those discharges that fall into the sample?**	Title

11. **Thank you for your time. I will be checking with you before I leave to say good-bye.**

At this time, could you introduce me to *(Names of person(s) listed in items 9a, 9b, 10a, and 10b).*

Notes

Figure I. Agency Questionnaire—Con.

OMB No. 0920-0298: Approval Expires 03/31/97

FORM **HHCS-3**
(3-29-96)

U.S. DEPARTMENT OF COMMERCE
BUREAU OF THE CENSUS
ACTING AS COLLECTING AGENT FOR THE
DEPARTMENT OF HEALTH AND HUMAN SERVICES
U.S. PUBLIC HEALTH SERVICE
CENTERS FOR DISEASE CONTROL AND PREVENTION
NATIONAL CENTER FOR HEALTH STATISTICS

CURRENT PATIENT QUESTIONNAIRE

1996 NATIONAL HOME AND HOSPICE CARE SURVEY

NOTICE – Public reporting burden for this collection of information is estimated to average 10 minutes per response, including the time for reviewing instructions, searching existing data sources, gathering and maintaining the data needed, and completing and reviewing the collection of information. Send comments regarding this burden estimate or any other aspect of this collection of information, including suggestions for reducing this burden to DHHS Reports Clearance Officer; Paperwork Reduction Project (0920-0298) Room 531-H; Hubert H. Humphrey Bldg.; 200 Independence Ave., SW; Washington, DC 20201. Information contained on this form which would permit identification of any individual or establishment has been collected with a guarantee that it will be held in strict confidence, will be used for purposes stated for this study, and will not be disclosed or released to others without the consent of the individual or establishment in accordance with Section 308(d) of the Public Health Service Act (42 USC 242m).

Section A – ADMINISTRATIVE INFORMATION

1. Field representative name	**2.** FR code	**3.** Date of interview Month/Day/Year
		/　　/

Section B – PATIENT INFORMATION

1. Patient name or other identifier First　　　　　　M.I.　　Last	**2.** Patient line number

Section C – STATUS OF INTERVIEW

01 ☐ Complete
02 ☐ Partial
03 ☐ Patient included in sampling list in error
04 ☐ Incorrect sample line number selected
05 ☐ Refused
06 ☐ Assessment only
07 ☐ Unable to locate record
08 ☐ Less than 6 patients selected
09 ☐ Other noninterview – *Specify* _____
10 ☐ No current patients

NOTES

Figure II. Current Patient Questionnaire

Read to each new respondent.

In order to obtain national level data about the patients of hospices and home health agencies such as this one, we are collecting information about a sample of current patients. I will be asking questions about the background, health status, treatment, social contacts, and billing information for each sampled patient.

The information you provide will be held in strict confidence and will be used ONLY by persons involved in the survey and only for the purposes of the survey.

In answering these questions, it is especially important to locate the information in the patient's medical record. Do you have the medical file(s) and record(s) for *(Read name(s) of selected current patient(s))***?**

If not, ask the respondent to get it/them prior to beginning the interview. Fill sections A and B on the front of all the current patient forms while the respondent gets the records. If no record is available for a patient, try to obtain as much information as possible from whatever administrative records are available and/or from the respondent's memory.

---

1. What is . . .'s sex?

01 ☐ Male
02 ☐ Female

---

2. What is . . .'s date of birth?

Age (at admission)

Month	Day	Year

OR _____ Years OR _____ Months

HAND FLASHCARD 1.

3a. Which of these best describes . . .'s race?

Mark (X) only one box.

01 ☐ White
02 ☐ Black
03 ☐ American Indian, Eskimo, Aleut
04 ☐ Asian, Pacific Islander
05 ☐ Other – *Specify* _____
06 ☐ Don't know

---

b. Is . . . of Hispanic origin?

01 ☐ Yes
02 ☐ No
03 ☐ Don't know

---

4. What is . . .'s current marital status?

Mark (X) only one box.

01 ☐ Married
02 ☐ Widowed
03 ☐ Divorced
04 ☐ Separated
05 ☐ Never married
06 ☐ Single
07 ☐ Don't know

HAND FLASHCARD 2.

5a. Where is . . . currently living?

Mark (X) only one box.

01 ☐ Private residence
02 ☐ Rented room, boarding house
03 ☐ Retirement home
04 ☐ Board and care assisted living or residential care facility
05 ☐ Other type of health facility (including mental health facility) – *SKIP to item 6 Introduction*
06 ☐ Other – *Specify* ↙

_____

---

b. Is . . . living with family members, nonfamily members, both family and nonfamily members, or alone?

01 ☐ With family members
02 ☐ With nonfamily members
03 ☐ With both family members and nonfamily members
04 ☐ Alone
05 ☐ Don't know

FORM HHCS-3 (3-29-96)   Page 3

Figure II. Current Patient Questionnaire—Con.

Read the introductory paragraph for the Social Security Number only once for each respondent.

As part of this survey, we would like to have . . .'s Social Security Number. Provision of this number is voluntary and providing or not providing the number will have no effect in any way on . . .'s benefits. This number will be useful in conducting future followup studies. It will be used to match against the vital statistics records maintained by the National Center for Health Statistics. This information is collected under the authority of Section 306 of the Public Health Service Act.

6. **What is . . .'s Social Security Number?**	Social Security Number ☐☐☐ – ☐☐ – ☐☐☐☐ 01 ☐ Refused 02 ☐ Don't know
HAND FLASHCARD 3. 7. **Who referred . . . to this agency?** *Mark (X) all that apply.* *PROBE:* **Any other sources?**	01 ☐ Self/Family 02 ☐ Nursing home 03 ☐ Hospital 04 ☐ Physician 05 ☐ Health department 06 ☐ Social service agency 07 ☐ Home health agency 08 ☐ Hospice 09 ☐ Religious organization 10 ☐ Other – *Specify* _____ 11 ☐ Don't know
8. **What was the date of . . .'s most recent admission with your agency, that is, the date on which . . . was admitted for the current episode of care?**	Month Day Year ☐☐ ☐☐ ☐☐ 00 ☐ Only an assessment was done for this patient (patient was not provided services by this agency)
9a. **According to . . .'s medical record, what were the primary and other diagnoses at the time of that (admission/assessment)?** *PROBE:* **Any other diagnoses?**	00 ☐ No diagnosis Primary: 1 _____ Others: 2 _____ 3 _____ 4 _____ 5 _____ 6 _____
*Refer to Q8. If **ONLY** an assessment was done for this patient, END THE INTERVIEW AND COMPLETE SECTION C ON THE COVER. THEN GO TO the next current patient questionnaire.* *If the patient was admitted to the agency and provided services by the agency, CONTINUE this interview.* b. **According to . . .'s medical records, what are . . .'s CURRENT primary and other diagnoses?** *PROBE:* **Any other diagnoses?**	00 ☐ No diagnosis 01 ☐ Same as 9a Primary: 1 _____ Others: 2 _____ 3 _____ 4 _____ 5 _____ 6 _____

FORM HHCS-3 (3-29-96)

Figure II. Current Patient Questionnaire—Con.

9c. According to . . .'s medical record, did . . . have any diagnostic or surgical procedures that were related to . . .'s admission to this agency?	00 ☐ No procedures 01 ☐ Yes 1 _____ 2 _____
10. What type of care is . . . currently receiving from your agency? Is it home health care or hospice care?	01 ☐ Home health care 02 ☐ Hospice care
11a. Does . . . have a primary caregiver (outside of this agency)?	01 ☐ Yes 02 ☐ No. . . . . . } *SKIP to item 12* 03 ☐ Don't know
b. Does . . . usually live with (his/her) primary caregiver?	01 ☐ Yes 02 ☐ No 03 ☐ Don't know
HAND FLASHCARD 5. **c. What is the relationship of the primary caregiver to . . .?** *Mark (X) only one box.*	01 ☐ Spouse 02 ☐ Parent 03 ☐ Child 04 ☐ Daughter-in-law/Son-in-law 05 ☐ Other relative – *Specify* _____ 06 ☐ Neighbor 07 ☐ Friend 08 ☐ Volunteer group 09 ☐ Other – *Specify* _____ 10 ☐ Don't know
HAND FLASHCARD 6. **12. Which of these aids does . . . currently use?** *Mark (X) all that apply.* *PROBE:* **Any other aids?**	00 ☐ No aids used 01 ☐ Bedside commode 02 ☐ Brace (any type) 03 ☐ Cane 04 ☐ Crutches 05 ☐ Dentures (full or partial) 06 ☐ Eyeglasses (including contact lenses) 07 ☐ Hearing aid 08 ☐ Hospital bed 09 ☐ Orthotics 10 ☐ Shower chair 11 ☐ Walker 12 ☐ Wheel chair – Manually operated 13 ☐ Wheel chair – Motorized 14 ☐ Other – *Specify* _____

NOTES

Figure II. Current Patient Questionnaire—Con.

For items 13a–14b, refer to item 12.	01 ☐ Yes
13a. Does . . . have any difficulty in seeing (when wearing glasses)?	02 ☐ No . . . . 03 ☐ Not applicable (e.g., comatose) . . } *SKIP to item 14a* 04 ☐ Don't know . . . .
HAND FLASHCARD 7. **b. Is . . .'s sight (when wearing glasses) partially, severely, or completely impaired as defined on this card?**	01 ☐ Partially impaired 02 ☐ Severely impaired 03 ☐ Completely lost, blind 04 ☐ Don't know
14a. Does . . . have any difficulty in hearing (when wearing a hearing aid)?	01 ☐ Yes 02 ☐ No . . . . 03 ☐ Not applicable (e.g., comatose) . . } *SKIP to item 15a* 04 ☐ Don't know . . . .
HAND FLASHCARD 8. **b. Is . . .'s hearing (when wearing a hearing aid) partially, severely, or completely impaired, as defined on this card?**	01 ☐ Partially impaired 02 ☐ Severely impaired 03 ☐ Completely lost, deaf 04 ☐ Don't know

15. *HAND FLASHCARD 9.*

*Ask questions 15a through 15k in **PART I FIRST**. As you ask each part of the question, PAUSE to allow the respondent time to refer to the flashcard. Mark (X) the "Yes" box for each item the respondent says the patient has in his/her home. Then, **GO TO PART II**, and ask the question for each item marked "Yes" in Part I.*

PART I   Which of the following items does . . . have in (his/her) home?

PART II   Does . . . receive assistance from your agency staff in caring for or using:

a. Oxygen, respiratory therapy equipment?

(1) Ventilator/Respirator . . . . 01 ☐ Yes	01 ☐ Yes	02 ☐ No	03 ☐ Don't know
(2) Liquid oxygen delivery system . . . . 01 ☐ Yes	01 ☐ Yes	02 ☐ No	03 ☐ Don't know
(3) Oxygen concentrator . . . . . . 01 ☐ Yes	01 ☐ Yes	02 ☐ No	03 ☐ Don't know
(4) Gaseous oxygen delivery system . . . . . . 01 ☐ Yes	01 ☐ Yes	02 ☐ No	03 ☐ Don't know
(5) Nebulizer . . . . 01 ☐ Yes	01 ☐ Yes	02 ☐ No	03 ☐ Don't know
(6) Humidifier . . . . 01 ☐ Yes	01 ☐ Yes	02 ☐ No	03 ☐ Don't know
(7) Suction equipment . . . . 01 ☐ Yes	01 ☐ Yes	02 ☐ No	03 ☐ Don't know
(8) Tracheostomy . . . . 01 ☐ Yes	01 ☐ Yes	02 ☐ No	03 ☐ Don't know

b. Intravenous therapy equipment?

(1) Peripheral catheter . . . . 01 ☐ Yes	01 ☐ Yes	02 ☐ No	03 ☐ Don't know
(2) Midline catheter . . . . 01 ☐ Yes	01 ☐ Yes	02 ☐ No	03 ☐ Don't know
(3) Central venous catheter (e.g. Hickman, Broviac, Porta-cath., etc.) . . . 01 ☐ Yes	01 ☐ Yes	02 ☐ No	03 ☐ Don't know
(4) Infusion pumps . . . . 01 ☐ Yes	01 ☐ Yes	02 ☐ No	03 ☐ Don't know

c. Decubitus ulcer prevention/treatment equipment?

(1) Air mattress/air fluidized bed . . . . 01 ☐ Yes	01 ☐ Yes	02 ☐ No	03 ☐ Don't know
(2) Foam mattress (egg-crate mattress) . . . . . 01 ☐ Yes	01 ☐ Yes	02 ☐ No	03 ☐ Don't know

d. Enteral nutrition equipment?

(1) Nasogastric tube . . . . 01 ☐ Yes	01 ☐ Yes	02 ☐ No	03 ☐ Don't know
(2) Gastrostomy/jejunostomy tube . . . . 01 ☐ Yes	01 ☐ Yes	02 ☐ No	03 ☐ Don't know
(3) Pump . . . . 01 ☐ Yes	01 ☐ Yes	02 ☐ No	03 ☐ Don't know

CONTINUED ON NEXT PAGE   ***CONTINUED ON NEXT PAGE***

FORM HHCS-3 (3-29-96)

Figure II. Current Patient Questionnaire—Con.

15.   PART I – Continued

Which of the following items does . . . have in (his/her) home?

e. Dialysis equipment?

(1) **Peritoneal Dialysis – Manual (continuous)** . . 01 ☐ Yes

(2) **Peritoneal Dialysis – Automated (intermittent/continuous cyclic)** . . . . 01 ☐ Yes

(3) **Peritoneal – unspecified** . . . . 01 ☐ Yes

(4) **Hemodialysis** . . . . 01 ☐ Yes

f. Blood glucose monitor? . . . . 01 ☐ Yes

g. Drainage devices? . . . . 01 ☐ Yes

(1) **Wound/bile duct/ureteral drainage catheter** . . 01 ☐ Yes

(2) **Foley catheter** . . . . 01 ☐ Yes

(3) **Intermittent bladder catheterization** . . . . . . 01 ☐ Yes

(4) **External urinary collection devices (e.g. condom catheter)** . . . . 01 ☐ Yes

(5) **Urostomy** . . . . 01 ☐ Yes

(6) **Ileostomy/Colostomy** . . . . 01 ☐ Yes

h. Protective restraints (e.g. vests, belts)? . . . . . . 01 ☐ Yes

i. Pediatric care? . . . . 01 ☐ Yes

(1) **Apnea monitor** . . . . 01 ☐ Yes

(2) **Phototherapy lights/equipment** . . . . 01 ☐ Yes

j. Prenatal uterine monitoring? . . . . 01 ☐ Yes

k. Other? – *Specify* _____ . . . . 01 ☐ Yes

---

15.   PART II – Continued

Does . . . receive assistance from your agency staff in caring for or using:

. . . . . 01 ☐ Yes . . . . 02 ☐ No . . . . 03 ☐ Don't know

. . . . . 01 ☐ Yes . . . . 02 ☐ No . . . . 03 ☐ Don't know

. . . . . 01 ☐ Yes . . . . 02 ☐ No . . . . 03 ☐ Don't know

. . . . . 01 ☐ Yes . . . . 02 ☐ No . . . . 03 ☐ Don't know

. . . . . 01 ☐ Yes . . . . 02 ☐ No . . . . 03 ☐ Don't know

. . . . . 01 ☐ Yes . . . . 02 ☐ No . . . . 03 ☐ Don't know

. . . . . 01 ☐ Yes . . . . 02 ☐ No . . . . 03 ☐ Don't know

. . . . . 01 ☐ Yes . . . . 02 ☐ No . . . . 03 ☐ Don't know

. . . . . 01 ☐ Yes . . . . 02 ☐ No . . . . 03 ☐ Don't know

. . . . . 01 ☐ Yes . . . . 02 ☐ No . . . . 03 ☐ Don't know

. . . . . 01 ☐ Yes . . . . 02 ☐ No . . . . 03 ☐ Don't know

. . . . . 01 ☐ Yes . . . . 02 ☐ No . . . . 03 ☐ Don't know

. . . . . 01 ☐ Yes . . . . 02 ☐ No . . . . 03 ☐ Don't know

. . . . . 01 ☐ Yes . . . . 02 ☐ No . . . . 03 ☐ Don't know

. . . . . 01 ☐ Yes . . . . 02 ☐ No . . . . 03 ☐ Don't know

. . . . . 01 ☐ Yes . . . . 02 ☐ No . . . . 03 ☐ Don't know

. . . . . 01 ☐ Yes . . . . 02 ☐ No . . . . 03 ☐ Don't know

. . . . . 01 ☐ Yes . . . . 02 ☐ No . . . . 03 ☐ Don't know

---

16.   Does . . . have any difficulty in controlling (his/her) bowels?

01 ☐ Yes
02 ☐ No
03 ☐ Not applicable (e.g. infant, has an ostomy)
04 ☐ Don't know

---

17.   Does . . . have any difficulty in controlling (his/her) bladder?

01 ☐ Yes
02 ☐ No
03 ☐ Not applicable (e.g. infant, has an indwelling catheter, has an ostomy)
04 ☐ Don't know

NOTES

FORM HHCS-3 (3-29-96)   Page 7

Figure II. Current Patient Questionnaire—Con.

	Yes	No	Don't know	Not applicable (e.g., patient is bedfast)
HAND FLASHCARD 10. **18.** Does . . . currently receive personal help from this agency in any of the following activities as defined on this card - - *Mark (X) one box for each activity.*				
a. Bathing or showering?	01 ☐	02 ☐	03 ☐	04 ☐
b. Dressing?	01 ☐	02 ☐	03 ☐	04 ☐
c. Eating?	01 ☐	02 ☐	03 ☐	04 ☐
d. Transferring in or out of beds or chairs?	01 ☐	02 ☐	03 ☐	04 ☐
e. Walking?	01 ☐	02 ☐	03 ☐	04 ☐
f. Using the toilet room?	01 ☐	02 ☐	03 ☐	04 ☐

	Yes	No	Don't know	Not applicable (e.g., patient is bedfast)
HAND FLASHCARD 11. **19.** Does . . . receive personal help from your agency in any of the following activities – *Mark (X) one box for each activity.*				
a. Doing light housework?	01 ☐	02 ☐	03 ☐	04 ☐
b. Managing money?	01 ☐	02 ☐	03 ☐	04 ☐
c. Shopping for groceries or clothes?	01 ☐	02 ☐	03 ☐	04 ☐
d. Using the telephone (dialing or receiving calls)?	01 ☐	02 ☐	03 ☐	04 ☐
e. Preparing meals?	01 ☐	02 ☐	03 ☐	04 ☐
f. Taking medications?	01 ☐	02 ☐	03 ☐	04 ☐

HAND FLASHCARD 12.

20a. Which of these services does . . . currently receive **FROM YOUR AGENCY?**

Mark (X) all that apply.

PROBE: **Any other services?**

00 ☐ None
01 ☐ Continuous home care
02 ☐ Counseling
03 ☐ Homemaker-household services
04 ☐ Medications
05 ☐ Mental health services
06 ☐ Nursing services
07 ☐ Nutritionist services
08 ☐ Occupational therapy
09 ☐ Physical therapy
10 ☐ Physician services
11 ☐ Social services
12 ☐ Speech therapy/Audiology
13 ☐ Transportation
14 ☐ Volunteers
15 ☐ Other services – *Specify* ↙

_____

NOTES

HAND FLASHCARD 13.

20b. Which of these service providers FROM YOUR AGENCY visited . . . during the last 30 days?

Mark (X) all that apply.

PROBE: **Any other providers?**

00 ☐ None
01 ☐ Chaplain
02 ☐ Dieticians/Nutritionists
03 ☐ Home health aides
04 ☐ Homemakers/Personal caretakers
05 ☐ Licensed practical or vocational nurses
06 ☐ Nursing aides and attendants
07 ☐ Occupational therapists
08 ☐ Physical therapists
09 ☐ Physicians
10 ☐ Registered nurses
11 ☐ Respiratory therapists
12 ☐ Social workers
13 ☐ Speech pathologists/audiologists
14 ☐ Volunteers
15 ☐ Other providers – *Specify* ↙

_____

HAND FLASHCARD 14.

21. What is the PRIMARY expected source of payment for . . . 's care?

Mark (X) only one source.

For the source of payment ask:
Is the *(source of payment)* **for home health care or hospice care?**

	Home Health Care	Hospice Care
01 ☐ Private insurance	01 ☐	01 ☐
02 ☐ Own income, family support, Social Security benefits, retirement funds, or welfare	02 ☐	02 ☐
03 ☐ Supplemental Security Income (SSI)	03 ☐	03 ☐
04 ☐ Medicare	04 ☐	04 ☐
05 ☐ Medicaid	05 ☐	05 ☐
06 ☐ Other government medical assistance	06 ☐	06 ☐
07 ☐ Religious organizations, foundations, agencies	07 ☐	07 ☐
08 ☐ VA contract, pensions, or other VA compensation	08 ☐	08 ☐
09 ☐ No charge made for care	09 ☐	09 ☐
10 ☐ Payment source not yet determined	10 ☐	10 ☐
11 ☐ Other – *Specify* ↙	11 ☐	11 ☐

_____

12 ☐ Don't know

NOTES

Figure II. Current Patient Questionnaire—Con.

HAND FLASHCARD 14.

22. What are ALL the secondary sources of payment for . . . 's care?

Mark (X) all that apply.

PROBE: **Any other sources of payment?**

For the source of payment ask:
Is the *(source of payment)* **for home health care or hospice care?**

		Home Health Care	Hospice Care
01 ☐	Private insurance	01 ☐	01 ☐
02 ☐	Own income, family support, Social Security benefits, retirement funds, or welfare	02 ☐	02 ☐
03 ☐	Supplemental Security Income (SSI)	03 ☐	03 ☐
04 ☐	Medicare	04 ☐	04 ☐
05 ☐	Medicaid	05 ☐	05 ☐
06 ☐	Other government medical assistance	06 ☐	06 ☐
07 ☐	Religious organizations, foundations, agencies	07 ☐	07 ☐
08 ☐	VA contract, pensions, or other VA compensation	08 ☐	08 ☐
09 ☐	No charge made for care	09 ☐	09 ☐
10 ☐	Payment source not yet determined	10 ☐	10 ☐
11 ☐	Other – *Specify* ↙	11 ☐	11 ☐
12 ☐	Don't know		

23. When was the last time service was provided?

Month	Day	Year

FILL SECTION C ON THE COVER OF THIS FORM AND CONTINUE WITH THE NEXT CURRENT PATIENT QUESTIONNAIRE.

NOTES

☆U.S. GOVERNMENT PRINTING OFFICE: 1996 - 750-112/40034

FORM HHCS-3 (3-29-96)

Figure II. Current Patient Questionnaire—Con.

OMB No. 0920-0298: Approval Expires 03/31/97

FORM **HHCS-5**
(3-29-96)

U.S. DEPARTMENT OF COMMERCE
BUREAU OF THE CENSUS
ACTING AS COLLECTING AGENT FOR THE
DEPARTMENT OF HEALTH AND HUMAN SERVICES
U.S. PUBLIC HEALTH SERVICE
CENTERS FOR DISEASE CONTROL AND PREVENTION
NATIONAL CENTER FOR HEALTH STATISTICS

DISCHARGED PATIENT QUESTIONNAIRE

1996 NATIONAL HOME AND
HOSPICE CARE SURVEY

NOTICE – Public reporting burden for this collection of information is estimated to average 10 minutes per response, including the time for reviewing instructions, searching existing data sources, gathering and maintaining the data needed, and completing and reviewing the collection of information. Send comments regarding this burden estimate or any other aspect of this collection of information, including suggestions for reducing this burden to DHHS Reports Clearance Officer; Paperwork Reduction Project (0920-0298) Room 531-H; Hubert H. Humphrey Bldg.; 200 Independence Ave., SW; Washington, DC 20201. Information contained on this form which would permit identification of any individual or establishment has been collected with a guarantee that it will be held in strict confidence, will be used for purposes stated for this study, and will not be disclosed or released to others without the consent of the individual or establishment in accordance with Section 308(d) of the Public Health Service Act (42 USC 242m).

Section A – ADMINISTRATIVE INFORMATION

| **1.** Field representative name | **2.** FR code | **3.** Date of interview Month/Day/Year ___/___/___ |

Section B – PATIENT INFORMATION

| **1.** Patient name or other identifier First   M.I.   Last | **2.** Patient line number | **3.** Date of Discharge Month/Day/Year ___/___/___ |

Section C – STATUS OF INTERVIEW

01 ☐ Complete
02 ☐ Partial
03 ☐ Patient included in sampling list in error
04 ☐ Incorrect sample line number selected
05 ☐ Refused
06 ☐ Assessment only
07 ☐ Unable to locate record
08 ☐ Less than 6 discharges selected
09 ☐ Other noninterview – *Specify* _____
10 ☐ No discharges

NOTES

Figure III. Discharge Patient Questionnaire

Read to each new respondent.

In order to obtain national level data about patients who are discharged from hospices and home health agencies such as this one, we are collecting information about a sample of discharges. I will be asking questions about the background, health status, treatment, social contacts, and billing information for each sampled discharge.

The information you provide will be held in strict confidence and will be used ONLY by persons involved in the survey and only for the purposes of the survey.

In answering these questions, it is especially important to locate the information in the patient's medical record. Do you have the medical file(s) and record(s) for *(Read name(s) of selected discharged patient(s))***?**

If not, ask the respondent to get it/them prior to beginning the interview. Fill sections A and B on the front of all the discharged patient forms while the respondent gets the records. If no record is available for a patient, try to obtain as much information as possible from whatever administrative records are available and/or from the respondent's memory.

---

1.   What was . . .'s sex?

01 ☐ Male
02 ☐ Female

---

2.   What was . . .'s date of birth?

Age (at admission)

Month	Day	Year

OR _____ OR _____
        Years   Months

HAND FLASHCARD 1.

3a. Which of these best described . . .'s race?

Mark (X) only one box.

01 ☐ White
02 ☐ Black
03 ☐ American Indian, Eskimo, Aleut
04 ☐ Asian, Pacific Islander
05 ☐ Other – *Specify* _____
06 ☐ Don't know

---

b. Was . . . of Hispanic origin?

01 ☐ Yes
02 ☐ No
03 ☐ Don't know

---

4.   What was . . .'s marital status at the time of discharge?

Mark (X) only one box.

01 ☐ Married
02 ☐ Widowed
03 ☐ Divorced
04 ☐ Separated
05 ☐ Never Married
06 ☐ Single
07 ☐ Don't know

HAND FLASHCARD 2.

5a. During the episode of care that ended on *(date of discharge)***, where was . . . living?**

Mark (X) only one box.

01 ☐ Private residence
02 ☐ Rented room, boarding house
03 ☐ Retirement home
04 ☐ Board and care assisted living or residential care facility
05 ☐ Other type of health facility (including mental health facility) – *SKIP to Item 6 Introduction*
06 ☐ Other – *Specify*

_____

---

b. Was . . . living with family members, nonfamily members, both family and nonfamily members, or alone?

01 ☐ With family members
02 ☐ With nonfamily members
03 ☐ With both family members and nonfamily members
04 ☐ Alone
05 ☐ Don't know

Figure III. Discharge Patient Questionnaire—Con.

Read the introductory paragraph for the Social Security Number only once for each respondent.

As part of this survey, we would like to have . . .'s Social Security Number. Provision of this number is voluntary and providing or not providing the number will have no effect in any way on . . .'s benefits. This number will be useful in conducting future followup studies. It will be used to match against the vital statistics records maintained by the National Center for Health Statistics. This information is collected under the authority of Section 306 of the Public Health Service Act.

---

6. What was . . .'s Social Security Number?

Social Security Number

☐☐☐ – ☐☐ – ☐☐☐☐

01 ☐ Refused
02 ☐ Don't know

HAND FLASHCARD 3.

7. Who referred . . . to this agency?

Mark (X) all that apply.

PROBE: **Any other sources?**

01 ☐ Self/Family
02 ☐ Nursing home
03 ☐ Hospital
04 ☐ Physician
05 ☐ Health department
06 ☐ Social service agency
07 ☐ Home health agency
08 ☐ Hospice
09 ☐ Religious organization
10 ☐ Other – *Specify* _____
11 ☐ Don't know

---

8. What was the date of . . .'s admission for the period of care which ended on *(Date of discharge)*?

Month	Day	Year

00 ☐ Only an assessment was done for this patient (patient was not provided services by this agency)

9a. According to . . .'s medical record, what were the primary and other diagnoses at the time of . . .'s admission that ended with this (discharge/assessment)?

PROBE: **Any other diagnoses?**

00 ☐ No diagnosis

Primary: 1 _____

Others: 2 _____

3 _____

4 _____

5 _____

6 _____

Refer to Q8. If **ONLY** *an assessment was done for this patient, END THE INTERVIEW AND COMPLETE SECTION C ON THE COVER. THEN GO TO the next discharged patient questionnaire.*

If the patient was admitted to the agency and provided services by the agency, CONTINUE this interview.

b. According to . . .'s medical records, what were . . .'s primary and other diagnoses at the time of discharge – that is, on *(Date of discharge)*?

PROBE: **Any other diagnoses?**

00 ☐ No diagnosis
01 ☐ Same as 9a

Primary: 1 _____

Others: 2 _____

3 _____

4 _____

5 _____

6 _____

Figure III. Discharge Patient Questionnaire—Con.

9c. According to . . .'s medical record, did . . . have any diagnostic or surgical procedures that were related to . . .'s admission to this agency?	00 ☐ No procedures 01 ☐ Yes 1 _____ 2 _____

HAND FLASHCARD 4.
 	
d. Why was . . . discharged?
 	
Mark (X) only one box.
 	
If the respondent answers "01 – Goals met", PROBE to determine which of the boxes "02–06" you should mark.
	01 ☐ Goals met
	     02 ☐ Recovered
	     03 ☐ Stabilized
	     04 ☐ Family/friends resumed care
	     05 ☐ Services no longer needed
	     06 ☐ Other – *Specify* _____
	
	07 ☐ Moved out of area
	08 ☐ Admitted to hospital
	09 ☐ Admitted to nursing home
	10 ☐ Benefits exhausted
	11 ☐ Charged/transferred home health/hospice agency
	12 ☐ Deceased
	13 ☐ Other – *Specify* _____
	14 ☐ Don't know

10. What type of care was . . . receiving at the time of discharge? Was it home health care or hospice care?	01 ☐ Home health care 02 ☐ Hospice care
11a. Did . . . have a primary caregiver (outside of this agency)?	01 ☐ Yes 02 ☐ No . . . . . . } *SKIP to item 12* 03 ☐ Don't know } *INSTRUCTION BOX*
b. Did . . . usually live with (his/her) primary caregiver?	01 ☐ Yes 02 ☐ No 03 ☐ Don't know
HAND FLASHCARD 5. **c. What was the relationship of the primary caregiver to . . .?** *Mark (X) only one box.*	01 ☐ Spouse 02 ☐ Parent 03 ☐ Child 04 ☐ Daughter-in-law/Son-in-law 05 ☐ Other relative – *Specify* _____ 06 ☐ Neighbor 07 ☐ Friend 08 ☐ Volunteer group 09 ☐ Other – *Specify* _____ 10 ☐ Don't know
INSTRUCTION BOX	*For items 12 through 19, use the phrase* "THE LAST TIME SERVICE WAS PROVIDED PRIOR TO (discharge on *date of discharge*)" *if the patient was discharged alive. Use the phrase* "THE LAST TIME SERVICE WAS PROVIDED PRIOR TO (death)" *if the patient was discharged dead.*
HAND FLASHCARD 6. **12.** The following questions refer to the patient's status the last time service was provided prior to **(discharge on** *date of discharge***/death).** The last time service was provided prior to **(discharge on** *date of discharge***/death), which of these aids did . . . regularly use?** *Mark (X) all that apply.* *PROBE:* **Any other aids?**	00 ☐ No aids used 01 ☐ Bedside commode 02 ☐ Brace (any type) 03 ☐ Cane 04 ☐ Crutches 05 ☐ Dentures (full or partial) 06 ☐ Eyeglasses (including contact lenses) 07 ☐ Hearing aid 08 ☐ Hospital bed 09 ☐ Orthotics 10 ☐ Shower chair 11 ☐ Walker 12 ☐ Wheel chair – Manually operated 13 ☐ Wheel chair – Motorized 14 ☐ Other – *Specify* _____

Figure III. Discharge Patient Questionnaire—Con.

For items 13a–14b, refer to item 12.	01 ☐ Yes
13a. The last time service was provided prior to (discharge on *date of discharge*/**death), did . . . have any difficulty in seeing (when wearing glasses)?**	02 ☐ No . . . . ⎫ 03 ☐ Not applicable (e.g., comatose) . . ⎬ *SKIP to item 14a* 04 ☐ Don't know . . . . ⎭
HAND FLASHCARD 7. **b. Was . . .'s sight (when wearing glasses) partially, severely, or completely impaired as defined on this card?**	01 ☐ Partially impaired 02 ☐ Severely impaired 03 ☐ Completely lost, blind 04 ☐ Don't know
14a. The last time service was provided prior to (discharge on *date of discharge*/**death), did . . . have any difficulty in hearing (when wearing a hearing aid)?**	01 ☐ Yes 02 ☐ No . . . . ⎫ 03 ☐ Not applicable (e.g., comatose) . . ⎬ *SKIP to item 15a* 04 ☐ Don't know . . . . ⎭
HAND FLASHCARD 8. **b. Was . . .'s hearing (when wearing a hearing aid) partially, severely, or completely impaired, as defined on this card?**	01 ☐ Partially impaired 02 ☐ Severely impaired 03 ☐ Completely lost, deaf 04 ☐ Don't know

15. *HAND FLASHCARD 9.*

Ask questions 15a through 15k in **PART I FIRST***. As you ask each part of the question, PAUSE to allow the respondent time to refer to the flashcard. Mark (X) the "Yes" box for each item the respondent says the patient had in his/her home. Then,* **GO TO PART II***, and ask the question for each item marked "Yes" in Part I.*

PART I The following questions refer to the patient's status the last time service was provided prior to (discharge on *date of discharge*/death). The last time service was provided prior to (discharge on *date of discharge*/death), which of the following items did . . . have in (his/her) home?	**PART II** Did . . . receive assistance from your agency staff in caring for or using:

a. Oxygen, respiratory therapy equipment?

(1) Ventilator/Respirator . . . . 01 ☐ Yes	01 ☐ Yes	02 ☐ No	03 ☐ Don't know
(2) Liquid oxygen delivery system . . . . 01 ☐ Yes	01 ☐ Yes	02 ☐ No	03 ☐ Don't know
(3) Oxygen concentrator . . . . 01 ☐ Yes	01 ☐ Yes	02 ☐ No	03 ☐ Don't know
(4) Gaseous oxygen delivery system . . . . . . 01 ☐ Yes	01 ☐ Yes	02 ☐ No	03 ☐ Don't know
(5) Nebulizer . . . . 01 ☐ Yes	01 ☐ Yes	02 ☐ No	03 ☐ Don't know
(6) Humidifier . . . . 01 ☐ Yes	01 ☐ Yes	02 ☐ No	03 ☐ Don't know
(7) Suction equipment . . . . 01 ☐ Yes	01 ☐ Yes	02 ☐ No	03 ☐ Don't know
(8) Tracheostomy . . . . 01 ☐ Yes	01 ☐ Yes	02 ☐ No	03 ☐ Don't know

b. Intravenous therapy equipment?

(1) Peripheral catheter . . . . 01 ☐ Yes	01 ☐ Yes	02 ☐ No	03 ☐ Don't know
(2) Midline catheter . . . . 01 ☐ Yes	01 ☐ Yes	02 ☐ No	03 ☐ Don't know
(3) Central venous catheter (e.g. Hickman, Broviac, Porta-cath., etc.) . . . . 01 ☐ Yes	01 ☐ Yes	02 ☐ No	03 ☐ Don't know
(4) Infusion pumps . . . . 01 ☐ Yes	01 ☐ Yes	02 ☐ No	03 ☐ Don't know

c. Decubitus ulcer prevention/treatment equipment?

(1) Air mattress/air fluidized bed . . . . 01 ☐ Yes	01 ☐ Yes	02 ☐ No	03 ☐ Don't know
(2) Foam mattress (egg-crate mattress) . . . . . 01 ☐ Yes	01 ☐ Yes	02 ☐ No	03 ☐ Don't know

d. Enteral nutrition equipment?

(1) Nasogastric tube . . . . 01 ☐ Yes	01 ☐ Yes	02 ☐ No	03 ☐ Don't know
(2) Gastrostomy/jejunostomy tube . . . . 01 ☐ Yes	01 ☐ Yes	02 ☐ No	03 ☐ Don't know
(3) Pump . . . . 01 ☐ Yes	01 ☐ Yes	02 ☐ No	03 ☐ Don't know

CONTINUED ON NEXT PAGE	*CONTINUED ON NEXT PAGE*

FORM HHCS-5 (3-29-96)

Figure III. Discharge Patient Questionnaire—Con.

15. **PART I – Continued**	15. **PART II – Continued**

The last time service was provided prior to (discharge on *date of discharge*/death), which of the following items did . . . have in (his/her) home?

Did . . . receive assistance from your agency staff in caring for or using:

e. **Dialysis equipment?**

　(1) **Peritoneal Dialysis – Manual (continuous)** . . 01 ☐ Yes　. . . . . 01 ☐ Yes　. . . . 02 ☐ No　. . . . 03 ☐ Don't know

　(2) **Peritoneal Dialysis – Automated (intermittent/continuous cyclic)** . . . . 01 ☐ Yes　. . . . . 01 ☐ Yes　. . . . 02 ☐ No　. . . . 03 ☐ Don't know

　(3) **Peritoneal – unspecified** . . . . 01 ☐ Yes　. . . . . 01 ☐ Yes　. . . . 02 ☐ No　. . . . 03 ☐ Don't know

　(4) **Hemodialysis** . . . . 01 ☐ Yes　. . . . . 01 ☐ Yes　. . . . 02 ☐ No　. . . . 03 ☐ Don't know

f. **Blood glucose monitor?** . . . . 01 ☐ Yes　. . . . . 01 ☐ Yes　. . . . 02 ☐ No　. . . . 03 ☐ Don't know

g. **Drainage devices?** . . . . 01 ☐ Yes　. . . . . 01 ☐ Yes　. . . . 02 ☐ No　. . . . 03 ☐ Don't know

　(1) **Wound/bile duct/ureteral drainage catheter** . . 01 ☐ Yes　. . . . . 01 ☐ Yes　. . . . 02 ☐ No　. . . . 03 ☐ Don't know

　(2) **Foley catheter** . . . . 01 ☐ Yes　. . . . . 01 ☐ Yes　. . . . 02 ☐ No　. . . . 03 ☐ Don't know

　(3) **Intermittent bladder catheterization** . . . . . . 01 ☐ Yes　. . . . . 01 ☐ Yes　. . . . 02 ☐ No　. . . . 03 ☐ Don't know

　(4) **External urinary collection devices (e.g. condom catheter)** . . . . 01 ☐ Yes　. . . . . 01 ☐ Yes　. . . . 02 ☐ No　. . . . 03 ☐ Don't know

　(5) **Urostomy** . . . . 01 ☐ Yes　. . . . . 01 ☐ Yes　. . . . 02 ☐ No　. . . . 03 ☐ Don't know

　(6) **Ileostomy/Colostomy** . . . . 01 ☐ Yes　. . . . . 01 ☐ Yes　. . . . 02 ☐ No　. . . . 03 ☐ Don't know

h. **Protective restraints (e.g. vests, belts)?** . . . . . . 01 ☐ Yes　. . . . . 01 ☐ Yes　. . . . 02 ☐ No　. . . . 03 ☐ Don't know

i. **Pediatric care?** . . . . 01 ☐ Yes　. . . . . 01 ☐ Yes　. . . . 02 ☐ No　. . . . 03 ☐ Don't know

　(1) **Apnea monitor** . . . . 01 ☐ Yes　. . . . . 01 ☐ Yes　. . . . 02 ☐ No　. . . . 03 ☐ Don't know

　(2) **Phototherapy lights/equipment** . . . . 01 ☐ Yes　. . . . . 01 ☐ Yes　. . . . 02 ☐ No　. . . . 03 ☐ Don't know

j. **Prenatal uterine monitoring?** . . . . 01 ☐ Yes　. . . . . 01 ☐ Yes　. . . . 02 ☐ No　. . . . 03 ☐ Don't know

k. **Other?** – *Specify* _____ . . . . 01 ☐ Yes　. . . . . 01 ☐ Yes　. . . . 02 ☐ No　. . . . 03 ☐ Don't know

---

16. The last time service was provided prior to (discharge on *date of discharge*/death), did . . . have any difficulty in controlling (his/her) bowels?

01 ☐ Yes
02 ☐ No
03 ☐ Not applicable (e.g. infant, had an ostomy)
04 ☐ Don't know

---

17. The last time service was provided prior to (discharge on *date of discharge*/death), did . . . have any difficulty in controlling (his/her) bladder?

01 ☐ Yes
02 ☐ No
03 ☐ Not applicable (e.g. infant, had an indwelling catheter, had an ostomy)
04 ☐ Don't know

NOTES

Figure III. Discharge Patient Questionnaire—Con.

HAND FLASHCARD 10.	Yes	No	Don't know	Not applicable (e.g., patient was bedfast)
18. The last time service was provided prior to (discharge on _date of discharge/_**death), did . . . receive personal help from this agency in any of the following activities as defined on this card - -** _Mark (X) one box for each activity._				
a. **Bathing or showering?**	01 ☐	02 ☐	03 ☐	04 ☐
b. **Dressing?**	01 ☐	02 ☐	03 ☐	04 ☐
c. **Eating?**	01 ☐	02 ☐	03 ☐	04 ☐
d. **Transferring in or out of beds or chairs?**	01 ☐	02 ☐	03 ☐	04 ☐
e. **Walking?**	01 ☐	02 ☐	03 ☐	04 ☐
f. **Using the toilet room?**	01 ☐	02 ☐	03 ☐	04 ☐
HAND FLASHCARD 11.	Yes	No	Don't know	Not applicable (e.g., patient was bedfast)
19. The last time service was provided prior to (discharge on _date of discharge/_**death), did . . . receive personal help from your agency in any of the following activities –** _Mark (X) one box for each activity._				
a. **Doing light housework?**	01 ☐	02 ☐	03 ☐	04 ☐
b. **Managing money?**	01 ☐	02 ☐	03 ☐	04 ☐
c. **Shopping for groceries or clothes?**	01 ☐	02 ☐	03 ☐	04 ☐
d. **Using the telephone (dialing or receiving calls)?**	01 ☐	02 ☐	03 ☐	04 ☐
e. **Preparing meals?**	01 ☐	02 ☐	03 ☐	04 ☐
f. **Taking medications?**	01 ☐	02 ☐	03 ☐	04 ☐

HAND FLASHCARD 12.

20a. During the 30 days prior to discharge, which of these services were provided to . . . BY YOUR AGENCY?

Mark (X) all that apply.

PROBE: **Any other services?**

00 ☐ None
01 ☐ Continuous home care
02 ☐ Counseling
03 ☐ Homemaker-household services
04 ☐ Medications
05 ☐ Mental health services
06 ☐ Nursing services
07 ☐ Nutritionist services
08 ☐ Occupational therapy
09 ☐ Physical therapy
10 ☐ Physician services
11 ☐ Social services
12 ☐ Speech therapy/Audiology
13 ☐ Transportation
14 ☐ Volunteers
15 ☐ Other services – _Specify_ ↙

_____

NOTES

　　　　　　　　　　　　　　　　　　FORM HHCS-5 (3-29-96)

Figure III. Discharge Patient Questionnaire—Con.

HAND FLASHCARD 13.

20b. During the 30 days prior to discharge, which of these service providers FROM YOUR AGENCY visited . . .?

Mark (X) all that apply.

PROBE: **Any other providers?**

00 ☐ None
01 ☐ Chaplain
02 ☐ Dieticians/Nutritionists
03 ☐ Home health aides
04 ☐ Homemakers/Personal caretakers
05 ☐ Licensed practical or vocational nurses
06 ☐ Nursing aides and attendants
07 ☐ Occupational therapists
08 ☐ Physical therapists
09 ☐ Physicians
10 ☐ Registered nurses
11 ☐ Respiratory therapists
12 ☐ Social workers
13 ☐ Speech pathologists/audiologists
14 ☐ Volunteers
15 ☐ Other providers – *Specify* ↗

_____

HAND FLASHCARD 14.

21. What was the PRIMARY expected source of payment for . . . 's entire episode of care?

Mark (X) only one source.

For the source of payment ask:
Was the *(source of payment)* **for home health care or hospice care?**

	Home Health Care	Hospice Care
01 ☐ Private insurance	01 ☐	01 ☐
02 ☐ Own income, family support, Social Security benefits, retirement funds, or welfare	02 ☐	02 ☐
03 ☐ Supplemental Security Income (SSI)	03 ☐	03 ☐
04 ☐ Medicare	04 ☐	04 ☐
05 ☐ Medicaid	05 ☐	05 ☐
06 ☐ Other government medical assistance	06 ☐	06 ☐
07 ☐ Religious organizations, foundations, agencies	07 ☐	07 ☐
08 ☐ VA contract, pensions, or other VA compensation	08 ☐	08 ☐
09 ☐ No charge made for care	09 ☐	09 ☐
10 ☐ Payment source not yet determined	10 ☐	10 ☐
11 ☐ Other – *Specify* ↗	11 ☐	11 ☐

_____

12 ☐ Don't know

NOTES

FORM HHCS-5 (3-29-96)

Page 9

Figure III. Discharge Patient Questionnaire—Con.

HAND FLASHCARD 14.

		Home Health Care	Hospice Care
22. **What were ALL the secondary sources of payment for . . . 's entire episode of care?**	01 ☐ Private insurance	01 ☐	01 ☐
Mark (X) all that apply.	02 ☐ Own income, family support, Social Security benefits, retirement funds, or welfare	02 ☐	02 ☐
PROBE: **Any other sources of payment?**	03 ☐ Supplemental Security Income (SSI)	03 ☐	03 ☐
For the source of payment ask: **Was the** *(source of payment)* **for home health care or hospice care?**	04 ☐ Medicare	04 ☐	04 ☐
	05 ☐ Medicaid	05 ☐	05 ☐
	06 ☐ Other government medical assistance	06 ☐	06 ☐
	07 ☐ Religious organizations, foundations, agencies	07 ☐	07 ☐
	08 ☐ VA contract, pensions, or other VA compensation	08 ☐	08 ☐
	09 ☐ No charge made for care	09 ☐	09 ☐
	10 ☐ Payment source not yet determined	10 ☐	10 ☐
	11 ☐ Other – *Specify* ↘	11 ☐	11 ☐
	12 ☐ Don't know		

23. When was the last time service was provided?

Month	Day	Year

**FILL SECTION C ON THE COVER OF THIS FORM AND CONTINUE
WITH THE NEXT DISCHARGED PATIENT QUESTIONNAIRE.**

NOTES

☆U.S. GOVERNMENT PRINTING OFFICE: 1996 - 750-112/40033

FORM HHCS-5 (3-29-96)

Figure III. Discharge Patient Questionnaire—Con.

Suggested citation

Haupt BJ. An overview of home health and
hospice care patients: 1996 National Home
and Hospice Care Survey. Advance data from
vital and health statistics; no. 297. Hyattsville,
Maryland: National Center for Health
Statistics. 1998.

National Center for Health Statistics

Director
Edward J. Sondik, Ph.D.

Deputy Director
Jack R. Anderson

DEPARTMENT OF
HEALTH & HUMAN SERVICES

Centers for Disease Control and Prevention
National Center for Health Statistics
6525 Belcrest Road
Hyattsville, Maryland 20782-2003

OFFICIAL BUSINESS
PENALTY FOR PRIVATE USE, $300

To receive this publication regularly, contact
the National Center for Health Statistics by
calling 301-436-8500
E-mail: nchsquery@cdc.gov
Internet: www.cdc.gov/nchswww/

DHHS Publication No. (PHS) 98-1250
8-0419 (4/98)

FIRST CLASS MAIL
POSTAGE & FEES PAID
PHS/NCHS
PERMIT NO. G-281